T0270094

The
Good
Eater

The
Good
Eater

A Vegan's Search for
the Future of Food

Nina Guilbeault

BLOOMSBURY PUBLISHING
NEW YORK • LONDON • OXFORD • NEW DELHI • SYDNEY

BLOOMSBURY PUBLISHING
Bloomsbury Publishing Inc.
1385 Broadway, New York, NY 10018, USA

BLOOMSBURY, BLOOMSBURY PUBLISHING, and the Diana logo are trademarks of
Bloomsbury Publishing Plc

First published in the United States 2024

Copyright © Nina Guilbeault, 2024

All rights reserved. No part of this publication may be reproduced or transmitted
in any form or by any means, electronic or mechanical, including photocopying, recording,
or any information storage or retrieval system, without prior permission in writing
from the publishers.

Bloomsbury Publishing Plc does not have any control over, or responsibility for, any
third-party websites referred to or in this book. All internet addresses given in this book
were correct at the time of going to press. The author and publisher regret any inconvenience
caused if addresses have changed or sites have ceased to exist, but can accept no
responsibility for any such changes.

DISCLAIMER: The author and publisher disclaim, as far as the law allows, any liability
arising directly or indirectly from the use, or misuse, of the information contained in this
book. This book is primarily a work of history and cultural criticism that examines the rise of
veganism within the broader context of our food system. This book is not intended to be,
and should not be, used as guidance or advice in respect of any health or medical conditions
or lifestyle choices.

ISBN: HB: 978-1-63557-699-3; EBOOK: 978-1-63557-700-6

LIBRARY OF CONGRESS CATALOGING-IN-PUBLICATION DATA IS AVAILABLE

2 4 6 8 10 9 7 5 3 1

Typeset by Westchester Publishing Services
Printed and bound in the U.S.A.

To find out more about our authors and books visit www.bloomsbury.com and sign up
for our newsletters.

Bloomsbury books may be purchased for business or promotional use. For information
on bulk purchases please contact Macmillan Corporate and Premium Sales Department at
specialmarkets@macmillan.com.

For Dedushka

With each meal, we make choices that help or harm the planet. What shall I eat today? is a very deep question.

—THICH NHAT HANH

CONTENTS

Introduction

The Vegan Wave

A generation ago, hardly anyone knew the word "vegan," much less knew what it meant. For those who had heard of the term, the image it conjured was likely of a stereotypical black-clad, tattooed, pierced animal rights protester bloodying fur coats with red paint at a fashion show. Or maybe a hippie restaurant like the one in *Annie Hall*, where Alvy Singer orders a plate of "alfalfa sprouts and mashed yeast." Cue the unappetizing smell emanating from the bulk section of the health food store, where "soy milk" was sold as a chalky powder, and "veggie" burgers looked like something astronauts would grudgingly eat on a space mission.

But in the last decade, veganism has undergone an almost unimaginable cultural makeover. The word "vegan" is everywhere—there's the little V certifying your favorite brand of cookies, the "cruelty-free" label on lipstick made with fruit pigments, and the option to choose vegan "pleather" for the interior of the latest hybrid car. From refined to hole-in-the-wall, restaurants are declaring their commitment to animal-free menu options, from "beet tartare" at fine dining establishments to the McPlant burger.

The popular image of the herbivore is becoming less stigmatized, too. The stereotypical activist "vegangelizing" the animal cause to passersby has been eclipsed by the ethereal influencer posting the perfect avocado toast on social media. A seemingly endless line of celebrities credit "plant-based" diets as the secret behind their glowing skin or sudden weight loss, and world-class athletes praise their meat-free regimes for giving them an edge in performance.

The coffee shop down the street now offers a selection of "milks" made from plants: not only a much-improved version of the vintage soy, which actually resembles milk, but also almond, oat, coconut, and even hemp. Vegan burgers, which used to be found in the specialty or health foods sections of the grocery store, now compete for your attention at the meat counter. These products are made of peas, potatoes, fungi, or even seaweed, but through the magic of food science, they are now virtually indistinguishable from conventional animal products in blind taste tests.

Even a global pandemic didn't slow down this trend. While the meat industry struggled with record numbers of COVID-19 cases among its vulnerable slaughterhouse worker populations, plant-based companies ramped up production in the midst of ingredient shortages and supply chain disruptions, and their investors shelled out billions in capital despite the coronavirus choking global financial markets. In the pandemic year of 2020, more than $2 billion was invested in plant-based products, making up nearly half of all the capital invested in the sector in the last forty years.[1]

The venture capital enthusiasm for "alternative proteins" mirrors demands from consumers. In 2022, the U.S. retail market for plant-based foods was worth $8 billion, up 7 percent from 2021, despite a challenging economic climate.[2] The global market is expected to grow exponentially, reaching up to $95 billion worldwide by 2029.[3] While plant-based milk is now a staple in many households, there's a tremendous growth of interest in other food categories, too, especially alternatives for meat, cheese, and eggs. More than half of American households now purchase some kind of plant-based product, and the vast majority come back for more.[4]

Meanwhile, new technologies are transforming how we produce food, in ways unimaginable even a decade ago. Already, scientists are using novel bioengineering tools to make "cruelty-free" animal products, like milk and egg whites, some of which are already available for sale. The next decade will also see the debut of meat grown directly from animal cells—what advocates call "cultivated" or "cell-cultured" meat and detractors call "lab-grown" meat. Although the jury is still out on how accessible these products will be, in terms of both cost and availability at scale, if these companies succeed, we may witness a true paradigm shift in food as we know it.

These cultural currents—along with documentaries exposing the horrors of the factory farming and fishing industries, the nutritional benefits of whole food plant-based diets, and the havoc animal agriculture is wreaking on the planet—have led to a seismic shift. Whereas the numbers of strict vegetarians and vegans remains at about 5 percent of the U.S. population,[5] a quarter of Americans[6] and as many as half of Europeans[7] are cutting down on animal products for health and environmental reasons, and consumers want even more vegan options than are currently available. They might call themselves "flexitarian," forgoing meat on Mondays, eating "vegan before six" (in the words of the former New York Times food columnist Mark Bittman), or embracing the memorable words of the food writer Michael Pollan: "Eat food. Not too much. Mostly plants."

Clearly, veganism is no longer the niche subculture it used to be. Once in the shadows, it's now in the cultural limelight. That raises the question: What happened?

I'm not the person you might expect to tell the story of how veganism entered the mainstream. My parents weren't hippies, and I ate plenty of meat and dairy earlier in my life. I was born in the Soviet Union in a tiny country called Moldova, landlocked between Romania and Ukraine, to a modest family of Russian, Ukrainian, and Jewish origins. Growing up in the rubble of the collapse, we didn't have much choice about what to eat.

As a child, I remember hearing stories from my parents and grandparents about the long lines for basics like milk and bread. My father routinely woke before sunrise to stand in line for a jug of milk that he manually churned into cottage cheese. In the summers, my grandparents rented a trailer by the woods and foraged for mushrooms, not as a hobby, but out of necessity. As the days grew colder, they'd spend days canning, preserving, and carefully storing food for the long, harsh winters.

When I was seven years old, we won the golden ticket, a chance to try our luck at the (North) American Dream. After applying to various countries, we were accepted as immigrants to Canada, mostly because its immigration system selects for those with higher educational backgrounds, and both my parents had been working on doctorates in physics (they were forced to drop out when the Soviet Union collapsed). When the Iron Curtain was drawn back, it revealed a people hungry for the Western way of life, including its food, and our new life in Toronto meant a world of delicacies opened up to our inexperienced palates.

At the grocery store, I marveled at the seemingly endless array of fruit yogurts, whole aisles of potato chip bags, gigantic racks of barbecued ribs, sugary cereals, tubs of ice cream in every flavor, and muffins, pies and cakes made ready-to-eat. Costco, especially, left an impression: more food than I could ever imagine under one roof, and a fridge at home big enough to store it. I used to roam the aisles as my parents shopped, unable to fully comprehend the abundance before me. The cornucopia was a revelation, and we quickly adopted the Western diet without a second thought.

Yet like many immigrant families, we continued to eat the familiar foods of our homeland, and Russians don't shy away from meat and dairy. My taste buds still awaken to memories of borscht (beet soup) with smetana (sour cream), blini (crêpes), tvorog (cottage cheese), sirniki (cottage cheese pancakes), pelmeni (meat dumplings), plof (a meaty rice dish), kalbasa (sausage), and salati ("salads" made of potatoes, peas, pickles, eggs, ham, and mayonnaise). Russian food is an odd mix of peasant fare inspired by French cuisine, but in giant portions. My fondest memory is of a layered custard cake named after Napoleon, a treat my Babushka would make for special occasions.

That's why, when I was a teenager, we were shocked when my father suddenly announced that he wanted to become a vegetarian. My dad grew up in an obscure village in a country nobody had heard of, and yet for years, he had apparently harbored a desire to give up meat. When he took up yoga and meditation to deal with the intense pressures of immigrant life, he felt a kinship with the Indian philosophical principle of *ahimsa*, "nonviolence," which preaches vegetarianism. Odd pucks of faux meat appeared in our freezer, large tubs of mixed nuts filled the cupboards, and soon my dad was putting a weird green paste on his toast, which I found totally off-putting. (This was way before avocado toast became a trendy thing.)

Our Russian friends, of course, made fun of him, teasing him with remarks about loss of manliness and warning that he would never feel satiated again. My dad wasn't sure he'd manage the transition, but he decided to give it a try out of moral principle. My sister and I got on the bandwagon, mostly because we admired his convictions. My mother, as well as her parents (who lived with us, as in many immigrant families), eventually had no choice but to accept the dietary divide in our house, a Berlin Wall of opposing food ideologies. My poor Babushka now generously cooked two separate dinners.

For many years, my vegetarianism wasn't a big part of my identity. If anything, I gladly compensated for the lack of meat in my diet with a hearty serving of dairy—yogurt, ice cream, and especially cheese. My love affair with cheese blossomed when I went to France for the first time at seventeen. Like countless clichéd Francophiles before me, I strolled the Parisian streets sampling every funky and creamy concoction. Who would deny themselves such pleasures? My mother used to say, "Vegans don't enjoy living," and your average French person would wholeheartedly agree with her.

But as is often the case with big life changes, a personal tragedy unexpectedly shifted my attitude. At the time, I was a couple of years into my graduate program in sociology at Harvard University, and I decided, rebelliously, to ditch Cambridge for the south of France while I studied for my general exams. I bought a one-way ticket to Nice, where I rented a tiny studio apartment on the outskirts of the city. In between study sessions at the rocky beach, I strolled the streets of the Old Town and blissfully—for ignorance truly can be blissful—I enjoyed all the gelato, brie, and pastries I fancied.

Then, one day, my father called me. My grandfather's cancer had taken a turn for the worse. My beloved Dedushka was the wise old grandfather of storybooks. I had last seen him over winter break after he'd had a medical emergency over Novi God (the Russian New Year). Rather than celebrating, I spent the holiday cooking meals, shuttling between hospitals, and translating doctors' orders. I will never forget the dreary yellow of the walls, which contrasted so distinctly with my own feeling of vibrant health, while spending days in waiting rooms. We thought he'd turned a corner, but now, my father said over the phone, he was gone.

The loss of our Dedushka was devastating and yet, as those who have experienced grief know, sometimes a glimmer of hope emerges out of the darkness. My grandfather's passing was the catalyst that inspired me to research the link between diet and disease, something I had never bothered to do before. What I found rocked me to my core, offering a glimpse of another reality where my whole family might have made different food choices, and where my Dedushka might have enjoyed more years of good health.

I learned that nutritional research had long shown that those following a plant-based diet have significantly lower rates of mortality from major diseases,[8] lower body weight[9] (even compared to health-conscious meat-eaters),[10] and longer lifespans.[11] I learned that only 5 to 10 percent of cancers are attributable to genetic defects, which means that the vast majority of cancers are rooted in environmental and lifestyle factors.[12] That includes breast, prostate, colorectal, endometrial, gallbladder, and pancreatic cancers.[13] In fact, there is strong evidence to suggest that a diet of exclusively, or even mostly, whole plant foods can treat and even reverse disease, including cancer.[14]

In 2015, the International Agency for Research on Cancer (IARC), the cancer research branch of the World Health Organization (WHO), reviewed more than eight hundred scientific papers on cancer and declared that there is "sufficient evidence of carcinogenicity" of processed meats (bacon, salami, sausages, beef jerky, ham, and such)—putting them in the same category as tobacco smoking and asbestos. They also declared that unprocessed red meat (from cattle, pigs, sheep, horses, goats, and so on) is "probably carcinogenic to humans."[15] The IARC used the word "probably" since the evidence on the carcinogenicity of meat is based on observational studies. Meat does contain certain important nutrients—including protein, vitamin B_{12}, and zinc. But these important nutrients can also be obtained from a healthful diet of plant foods that have been shown to contain compounds that protect against cancer and other diseases.[16]

Whether or not dairy is carcinogenic is a hotly debated topic. There is evidence both for and against its consumption, depending on the type of cancer. One of the clear links is between consumption of dairy products and increased likelihood of prostate cancer, the type of cancer that took my grandfather's life.[17] The mechanism appears to be the hormone insulin-like growth factor 1 (IGF-1), which is present in both low-fat and high-fat dairy and is linked to the proliferation of prostate cancer cells.[18] In a study comparing meat eaters, vegetarians, and vegans, vegans were found to have the lowest levels of IGF-1, but otherwise normal hormonal levels. (Incidentally, vegan men were found to have higher testosterone, which builds muscles and increases sex drive—flipping the narrative around meat eating and virility.)[19]

How is it that this information was not widely known? It seemed purposefully obscured by powerful lobbies working on behalf of the food and pharmaceutical industries. Reporting by the Center for Responsive Politics has documented that the thirty food and beverage companies that spent the most on lobbying in 2020 collectively spent almost $40 million.[20] Meanwhile, a report published by a prestigious medical journal showed that from 1999 to 2018, the pharmaceutical and health product industries spent $4.7 billion, an average of $233 million per year, on lobbying the U.S. federal government, $414 million on contributions to presidential campaigns, and $877 million on state candidates and committees to influence health care laws, drug pricing, and regulation. In other words, both food and health care, like other big business, cast long shadows over the political landscape.[21]

It seemed diabolically unfair, and I wondered what other truths lay buried beneath these perverse incentives. As the prominent physician Dr. David Katz eloquently expresses:

> A food supply in which "junk" is a food group, willfully engineered to maximize eating for profit, is tolerated with no obvious outrage by either parents or health professionals. Waiting for silver bullets, we let a pernicious truth hide in plain sight, squandering the potential to eliminate some 80% of chronic disease and premature death, and at the same time devastating our aquifers, our climate, our economy, and the great treasure of this planet's biodiversity.[22]

That summer, I went down a rabbit hole. Slowly, I learned many disturbing truths about our food system, including the outsize impact of the animal agriculture industry on climate change and chronic disease. I educated myself about the overuse of antibiotics on factory farms, a potentially cataclysmic problem that creates treatment-resistant bacterial strains that could be a catastrophic blow to modern medicine.[23] Unlike many of the most zealous converts, I didn't embrace the vegan lifestyle overnight. For me, it was a gradual process, two steps forward, one step back, until one day I found myself on the other side of an impossible divide and could no longer ignore the consequences of what I put on my plate. Although my new knowledge couldn't save my grandfather, it forever changed my life.

When I came back to my graduate program that autumn, I declared to my professors that I wanted to understand how veganism, long a niche subculture, was turning into a mainstream movement. My well-meaning mentors objected, pointing out that if I wanted an academic job, I'd better pick a topic that would appeal to more than just vegans, still a tiny fraction of society. They were right, of course, but I ignored their objections. I couldn't imagine a topic more important than one that touched on many of the biggest social issues confronting my generation, including climate change, social justice, chronic disease, and food security. I could sense the vegan wave cresting, and I wanted to be there when it hit shore.

Eventually, my committee gave in, and I was lucky enough to secure funding to research this growing movement around the world. My research took me back to France, the epicenter of gastronomy; to Germany, the European leader of the vegan renaissance; to India, with its deep history of vegetarianism; and to Israel, where I lived in an urban ecological co-op and witnessed the incredible rise of veganism in that tiny, complex country. Eventually—maybe inevitably—I landed on the California coast, first in Los Angeles and eventually in the Bay Area, to study the epicenters of veganism in the United States. All told, I spent over five years doing fieldwork and interviewing (in three languages) hundreds of people at the forefront of this massive cultural shift.

On my travels, I met every kind of vegan there is. Righteous activists defending the lives of innocent animals. Iconic influencers embodying the aspirational, health-conscious vegan lifestyle on social media. Fitness gurus proving that plants can power ambitious athletic performance. Documentary filmmakers, authors, and podcasters spreading the word. Visionary founders revolutionizing food technology in Silicon Valley, and deep-pocketed investors supporting their mission to end animal agriculture.

At first, I was starry-eyed. I was especially inspired by the entrepreneurs, and even tempted once or twice to drop out of grad school and start a company that, I believed, could change the world. Academia has a politically incorrect term for this tendency: "going native." It means losing one's scholarly objectivity and embracing the worldview of one's research subjects, and it comes mostly from anthropology. "Be careful not to drink the vegan Kool-Aid," my adviser repeatedly warned, implying that I was at risk of joining some kind of cult. She probably sensed I was already a lost cause.

Yet as I broadened my network and dived deeper into the vegan community from all its angles, I began to sense some of its internal frictions surfacing, especially at the boundaries of my various vegan friend groups.

There were the animal rights activists I met in Boston, Paris, and Tel Aviv, who toiled in underpaid jobs at charities to save as many animal lives as they could, committed to raising consciousness and expanding the moral circle. There were my social media influencer friends in Los Angeles, who followed strict health-conscious diets and eschewed any processed foods. Perhaps most charismatic were my biotech enthusiast friends in the Bay Area, who started "alternative protein" companies they hoped could change meat itself. All these groups were under the umbrella of a movement to change the future of food, and yet many had different—and often opposing—ideas about how to get there.

To be perfectly honest, I didn't identify with the bleeding-heart activists. My concern for animals was mostly intellectual. It seemed obvious that it was morally wrong to cause suffering to sentient beings, especially if we didn't *need* to eat meat, but I wasn't the type to go out of my way to visit an animal sanctuary and hug a cow.

At the same time, I couldn't fully comprehend the moral calculus of my purely rational vegan friends either, those inspired by effective altruism. Many of them started companies to make products that could compete with animal agriculture. I felt fully aligned with their mission, and yet when I saw some of their products, I couldn't help but experience a pang of disappointment that, despite the claims on their packages, they couldn't necessarily be considered healthful, and an unhealthful diet is now responsible for more deaths globally than any other cause, including other lifestyle factors like smoking or lack of exercise.[24] Still, I told myself, even though these foodstuffs belonged to the category labeled "processed foods," they must be far better than the status quo factory-farmed items they were designed to replace.

For me, these tensions came to a head when, at last, I defended my dissertation and moved to the Bay Area to begin a postdoctoral fellowship at UC Berkeley's Sustainable Food Initiative, where I planned to turn my research into this book. There, I was surprised to meet many food movement advocates who were, to say the least, skeptical of the new vegan products on offer, if not downright derisive. To them, the Impossible Burger did not herald some Silicon Valley techno-utopia where we can have our meat and eat it too. In their view, some of these new products, made of genetically modified soy sprayed with herbicides, reinforced the very same values— efficiency, uniformity, and cheapness—that uphold our industrialized fast food system.

Others expressed skepticism of a movement that was turning a philosophy with ancient (and often radical) origins into a glamorized lifestyle. They argued that such a shift represents a tone-deaf ignorance of deep cultural traditions tied to humble beginnings all around the world and excludes those who have been eating plant staples for generations. They wanted a future in which we returned to our roots, and even right back to the land, where we grew our own food, ate seasonally and locally, and cooked our own meals rather than expecting corporations to feed us.

There were undeniable truths in all these points of view, and I found myself trying to reconcile them. I became increasingly frustrated by the exaggerated claims of CEOs who knew how to tell a good story but didn't, it seemed to me, take the time to think deeply about true systemic transformation. But I felt equally irritated by self-proclaimed food experts who were concerned only about "animal welfare," or about their personal health, rather than thinking about our collective responsibility to sentient beings and to our home, the earth. Many assumed that since animals have always been a source of food for human beings, there couldn't possibly be anything wrong with that anthropocentric equation.

Today, we're collectively waking up to the reality that the most pressing problems we face—deforestation, water shortage, loss of biodiversity, chronic diseases in developed nations, food insecurity in developing ones, antibiotic resistance, and even pandemics—are tied in some way to the large-scale industrial production of animal products. Even so, many unanswered questions remain. Can our concerns for the fates of animals be addressed through behavioral change alone? Can we shift the food system without sacrificing convenience, affordability, and taste? Is capitalism the only route to systemic transformation? Can veganism be reconciled with the realities of feeding a growing world population? Can veganism scale without sacrificing its values?

As I wrestled with these questions within myself, I realized that the journey at the center of this book wasn't only, as I had initially thought, about the transformation of a movement, but also about my own inner transformation. While the book is centered on the tales of those at the vanguard of veganism, as well as their critics, it's also about how meeting these change makers shifted my own views about the future of food, and it might just shift your own.

In these pages, you will discover the philosophical roots of veganism, which trace as far back as antiquity to famous advocates like Pythagoras, Leonardo da Vinci, Leo Tolstoy, and Gandhi. You will learn about the modern animal rights movement, and how the failure to raise consciousness led to a paradigm shift that changed culture. You will walk through the headquarters of Silicon Valley start-ups innovating the future of food through novel technologies, including "meat" made of plants and real meat made without slaughter. And you will get an insider's look into the wealthy "vegan mafia" bankrolling the whole enterprise.

You will learn the true meaning of regenerative agriculture, and learn why its advocates often critique veganism, and meet a farmer trying to balance her commitment to both philosophies. You will learn about the pathbreaking nutritional research showing the benefits of a plant-based diet for both health and longevity, and how chefs are making vegetables irresistible. And you will learn the often ignored yet essential radical roots of veganism, including in the African diaspora. Along the way, you will savor meals (and learn to make tofu from a tofu master) that will make you reflect on your own answer to the question that inspired this book: Is there truly an ethical way to eat?

My own journey to answer this question led me to an entirely different place than I initially expected. At the outset of the book, I had been a diehard vegan on a mission to convince others of the value of my perspective, yet one who came to it from the perch of a rigorous academic. At the end—well, that's part of the story you will read in these pages. For now, let's just say that my position is far more nuanced and complex today than I ever expected.

The Good Eater is a deeply researched story of the cultural transformation of veganism, and the change makers behind it. But it also turned out to be a personal account of my own search for how to eat, and my attempts at reconciling the different visions I've encountered along the way. It is my attempt to, as Rainer Maria Rilke advised the young poet and a mentor at UC Berkeley advised me, "Be patient toward all that is unsolved in your heart and try to love the questions themselves." This book is the story of the search for what a just, nourishing, and equitable food system could look like, and for my place in cultivating it.

Chapter One

Setting the Table

If man is seriously seeking to live a good life, the first thing from which he will abstain will always be the use of animal products because it involves the performance of an act which is contrary to the moral feeling—*killing*—and is called forth only by the greediness and the desire for delicious food.

—LEO TOLSTOY

There is no definitive beginning to the history of veganism, but one good place to start is the year 1944. In the midst of the most destructive war of the century, a British man named Donald Watson was trying to come up with a new word. He wanted it to evoke a lifestyle in harmony with the planet, nonhuman animals, and personal vitality. At first he entertained "benevore" and "sanivore" from the prefixes *bene-*, meaning "well," and *sani,-* "healthful." Not quite right, he thought. He then considered emphasizing the food to be avoided with "dairyban," but that seemed too hardline. The term "vitan" seemed plausible, evoking vitality. With a nod to French, he briefly considered "beaumangeur" ("good eater"), but nothing quite clicked.

It was his wife, Dorothy, who landed on the winner. She suggested combining the beginning and ending of the word "vegetarian": *veg-* + *-an* = *vegan*. The term made sense, since the Watsons saw "veganism" as a natural extension of the philosophy of vegetarianism, which espouses the nonconsumption of animal flesh for moral, health, environmental, and spiritual reasons. On a sunny Sunday in November, the Watsons and others met at the Attic Club in Holborn, London, to officially found the Vegan Society.

But why, if the Vegetarian Society had already existed in England for a century? The Watsons and their friends held a strong conviction that the definition of vegetarianism had become muddled. It had originally referred to a diet that excluded the use of animals in any form, but over time it widened to include those who still consumed eggs and dairy products, confounding the meaning. The first vegetarian cookbook, called *Kitchen Philosophy for Vegetarians*—published in 1847 and coinciding with the creation of the original society—included no animal products, and many of the founders of the Vegetarian Society avoided animal-based foods entirely. Yet some within the early society came to see these rules as too extreme. While a stricter diet was acknowledged as the ideal, the members felt it alienated those who could not go all the way. As the magazine editor for the society wrote, "We feel that the ideal position for vegetarians is abstinence from animal products, and that most of us are, like other reformers, in a transitional stage."[1]

In the early twentieth century, there was a lively discussion in *The Vegetarian Messenger*, the publication of the Vegetarian Society, about what the definition of "vegetarianism" should be. The editors invited correspondence, and Donald Watson wrote in. Watson was born in Yorkshire to the headmaster of a mining community and became a woodworker. As an adolescent, he witnessed the slaughter of pigs on his uncle's farm, which horrified him, and he decided to stop eating meat. In his twenties, he removed not only animal products but also cooked foods from his diet altogether. "I decided early this year to try what must, I think, be the last of all vegetarian experiments, that is, to live exclusively on raw fruit," he wrote in his journal. "My diet now consists of nuts, bananas, apples, and dates."

In December 1943, Watson was invited to give a talk on dairy at the Vegetarian Society. A summary of the lecture was published in *The Vegetarian Messenger* in March 1944, inspiring a lively debate about the place of dairy in a vegetarian diet. As often happens, the Society was split down the middle. The majority felt the group's efforts should be spent on "abolishing flesh eating," while the remainder felt it was nonsensical to focus only on flesh rather than abolishing the use of animals entirely. That minority subset, led by Watson, decided to split from the larger group, ultimately founding the Vegan Society. Its stated mission at the time was to "seek and end the use of animals by man for food, commodities, work, hunting, vivisection, and by all other uses involving exploitation of animal life by man."[2]

It was a difficult historical moment to start a cultural revolution. Wartime in Britain meant rationed gasoline and food, so the group could not meet frequently. More important, food shortages made it challenging to obtain enough calories to sustain a balanced vegan diet. The early vegans tried to trade their butter and lard rations for lentils and dried fruits, but their appeals were rejected on account of not being nutritionally equivalent. Many also ran into problems with B_{12} deficiency before the discovery that this essential vitamin, found in soil bacteria, is lacking in modern plant foods due to overwashing. It took a lot of trial and error, but over time the early pioneers figured out how to not only survive, but thrive on a diet made up exclusively of vegetables, fruits, grains, legumes, nuts, and seeds.

Eight decades later, the Vegan Society still exists. You may have seen its little "V" symbol that certifies vegan products at the grocery store. The group's stated mission, revised when it became a charity in 1979, defines veganism as "a philosophy and way of living which seeks to exclude—as far as is possible and practicable—all forms of exploitation of, and cruelty to, animals for food, clothing or any other purpose; and by extension, promotes the development and use of animal-free alternatives for the benefit of animals, humans and the environment. In dietary terms it denotes the practice of dispensing with all products derived wholly or partly from animals."[3]

———————

While the philosophy of veganism may have been codified in the twentieth century, its roots span back further in history. Modern food gurus love to debate about what our ancestors ate, whether a diet centered mostly on plants or one in which meat played a pivotal role. The truth is somewhere in the middle. We are omnivores capable of digesting a wide variety of foods, including plants, animals, and fungi, and throughout time and place, what we ate depended on the ecology of where we lived.[4] Still, in most regions our diets consisted mainly of fruits and vegetables, despite what modern "paleo" or "carnivore" diet advocates may claim. Although meat is undoubtedly a part of our evolutionary history, we ate far less meat, and less consistently, than we consume today.[5]

Evidence for our mostly herbivorous past is etched right into our bodies. Our flat teeth are ideal for grinding down vegetable matter, and our long digestive tract is designed to break down fiber, which is found only in plants. The bulk of our diet consisted of foraged berries, seeds, and mushrooms, and later, starches such as the early ancestors of corn, wheat, and potatoes, so "hunter-gatherers" would best be thought of as "gatherer-hunters" or "foragers."[6] Our closest evolutionary relatives, chimpanzees, eat a plant-predominant diet, supplemented with a small amount of meat for essential nutrients. Gorillas, more distantly related, follow an exclusively plant-based diet but do eat some insects.[7] Archeological evidence of early humanoids shows us that our ancestors began consuming grains some 150,000 years ago, and that previous reports emphasizing the importance of meat were likely exaggerated: we were simply getting a distorted picture until recent technological developments made it possible to detect ancient plant matter.[8]

Still, in part because of its rarity and the difficulty of obtaining it, meat symbolized wealth and abundance, as well as community and social belonging, and in many societies it still does today. With the rise of agriculture and the domestication of livestock, food became more steadily available, and we came to enjoy more of all types of it, including animal-based foods, than at any time before in our evolutionary history.

Ironically, the steadier availability of food allowed us, for the first time, to be selective about our diet, and to develop moral convictions about our choices. As the historian Colin Spencer writes in *The Heretic's Feast*, "A taboo can only flourish in a well-fed community, where people have enough leisure to reflect on the meaning of existence."[9] In that sense, the true history of vegetarianism can be traced to an imprecise historical moment when food became plentiful enough that it became possible to abstain from the consumption of animals out of moral principle.

Many early vegetarians were motivated by ethical or spiritual convictions tied to beliefs about living in harmony with the earth, our body, and the cosmos. In some cases, entire cultures were formed around such convictions. Vegetarianism is especially prominent in many South and East Asian religious traditions, which promote the practice of *ahimsa*. This ancient Sanskrit word means "nonharm" or "nonviolence," and the concept is a cornerstone of Hinduism, Buddhism, and Jainism. Jains are among the most rigorous vegetarians; many practice elaborate rituals to avoid causing unnecessary harm to even the tiniest creatures, such as sweeping the path before them as they walk to avoid stepping on insects, or eschewing root vegetables, which are perceived to die when uprooted.

In contrast to the East, the common thread in Western culture is a kind of anthropocentrism that assumes a hierarchy of animals with humans (we sometimes even forget we're animals ourselves) at the top. Yet even in the West, there have always been powerful thinkers challenging the status quo. One of the earliest known vegetarians was the mathematician Pythagoras; in fact, until the term "vegetarian" became common in the 1850s, an animal-free diet was known as the Pythagorean diet. Born in the sixth century B.C.E. on Samos, off the coast of modern-day Turkey, Pythagoras was influenced by his tutors: Polycrates, who believed that the soul is immortal and passes on to another body, human or nonhuman, at the time of death; and

Thales, who believed that all inanimate matter is imbued with divine consciousness. Historians have even speculated that Pythagoras may have reached India on his travels and been influenced by Eastern thought there.

Pythagoras came to believe that since all living things are conscious, eating the flesh of another animal is immoral. It's hard to say whether he avoided animal foods entirely, as ancient dietary records are rare and vague, but it would have been consistent with his unconventional and surprisingly progressive views, including allowing women to study in his schools and emphasizing the development of moral character. Yet despite his influence as a mathematician, the titans of Western philosophy who came after him—Socrates, Plato, and Aristotle—ignored his moral convictions. How different the Western world might be if we had looked to Pythagoras, not Plato, for our ideal of morality.

The idea of humans as superior to nonhuman animals became calcified in the Judeo-Christian tradition that followed. In the Bible, the first words of God to Adam and Eve are "Be fruitful, and multiply, and replenish the earth, and subdue it; have dominion over the fish of the sea, and over the fowl of the air, and over every living thing that moveth upon the earth" (Genesis 1:28). Yet, intriguingly, the very next thing God says is "Behold, I have given you every herb bearing seed and every tree, in the which is the fruit of a tree yielding seed; to you it shall be for meat" (1:29), a passage which has been interpreted by some Christian groups, including the Seventh-day Adventists, as clear evidence of the injunction to eat an entirely plant-based diet.

At the dawn of the Renaissance, when Copernicus began to question the centrality of humans in the universe and recognized that the earth revolved around the sun and not the other way around, the assumed dominance of humans vis-à-vis other life forms still remained unquestioned. Even here, though, we find another naysayer, the Renaissance Man himself, Leonardo da Vinci. His studies of anatomy led him to realize that nonhuman animals, too, can feel pain. This insight led him to adopt what he called a "simple" diet of only vegetables and to wear linen so as not to, as a friend wrote about him, "wear something dead."[10] Da Vinci also routinely freed caged birds at the market. A friend wrote that "he would not kill a flea for any reason whatsoever."

While we have only scarce evidence of da Vinci's diet, what sources we do have point to his staunch vegetarianism. Writing from India to da Vinci's patron, Giuliano de' Medici, an explorer reported that the people there "do not feed on anything that has blood, nor will they allow anyone to hurt any living thing, like our dear Leonardo da Vinci." In his own journal, da Vinci wrote, "If you [humans] are, as you have described yourself, the king of the animals, why do you help other animals only so that they may be able to give you their young in order to gratify your palate?"[11] Today we celebrate da Vinci as an inventor, engineer, and artist, but just as with Pythagoras, we ignore his moral philosophy.

This cultural attitude continued into the Age of Enlightenment. This period saw revolutionary scientific discoveries and transformative new political philosophies, such as the notion that all men (at least white, wealthy, European men, only later all humans) are created equal. But the Enlightenment did not extend the moral circle beyond humanity. An important debate during this period was whether or not animals had "souls," meaning consciousness and the capacity to suffer. René Descartes, the most influential philosopher of his time, famously declared, "I think, therefore I am." By this, Descartes meant that his self-awareness of his own thinking proved that he was in fact conscious. Descartes did not, however, extend the same assumption of self-awareness to animals, and in fact he argued that animals were not conscious at all and therefore could not feel pain.

The Cartesian idea of a "clockwork universe," in which nonhuman animals are little more than unconscious automatons, appealed to many thinkers, who found it more convenient than the notion of dominion, which implied a kind of caretaking responsibility over the animal kingdom. The idea also fitted neatly with technological advances that made the cultivation and distribution of larger quantities of meat and other animal products possible. Animals became commodities, no different from any other manufactured products, ripe for technological innovation, optimization, and mechanization. The Industrial Revolution ratcheted animal agriculture into high gear, and the greater availability of animal products slowly changed the Western diet.

The upper classes in Europe began eating larger portions of meat than ever before, and it began to show. Wealthy people started to get sick from chronic diseases such as obesity and gout, and critics worried that excessive consumption by the rich would mean the poor would starve, since animal products took far more resources to produce than they yielded in food. In *A Modest Proposal*, the satirist Jonathan Swift facetiously suggested that, to solve this problem, the children of the poor be fed to the upper classes. His bitter indictment of absurd wealth inequality can also be read as a commentary on our relationship to the lowest of the low—the animals we believe exist for our consumption.

Yet once again, throughout the Industrial Revolution there were influential advocates of the vegetarian cause, including the writers Percy Bysshe Shelley, George Bernard Shaw, and Leo Tolstoy. Although Tolstoy is best known for his fiction masterpieces, *War and Peace* and *Anna Karenina*, in the second half of his life he had a spiritual awakening (his wife, Sonya, saw it as a "nervous breakdown") and began to write feverishly about progressive causes, including the education of serfs, pacifism, and the renunciation of hunting, alcohol, and meat. Tolstoy believed that vegetarianism suppressed lust and brought one closer to a higher spiritual calling, and as usual, the great Russian author did not mince words. Recounting a visit to an abattoir in the late 1890s, Tolstoy went into graphic detail describing how a cow is dismembered and how its blood trickles onto the killing floor. "We cannot pretend that we do not know this," he wrote. "We are not ostriches and cannot believe that if we refuse to look at what we do not wish to see, it will not exist. This is especially the case when what we do not wish to see is what we wish to eat."

Despite his personal failure to live up to his own ideals (he never managed to maintain a vegetarian diet for long),[12] Tolstoy's ideas influenced many later thinkers, among them Dr. Martin Luther King Jr., the philosopher Ludwig Wittgenstein, and a young lawyer named Mohandas Karamchand Gandhi. When the man who eventually became Mahatma Gandhi first embarked for England to study law in the 1880s, he promised his mother that he would avoid "women, wine, and meat."[13] But maintaining a purely vegetarian diet proved challenging in the cold and rainy metropolis. Faced with racism and pangs of hunger, Gandhi guiltily began eating meat, until one day he stumbled into a restaurant run by the London Vegetarian Society. The existence of the restaurant and its library of books by Tolstoy and others inspired Gandhi to return to his childhood regimen, a vegetarian diet rooted in the ancient culture he had inherited.

"When I went to England, I was a votary of violence, I had faith in it and none in nonviolence. After reading Tolstoy, that lack of faith in nonviolence vanished,"[14] Gandhi wrote, drawing a direct link between his diet and politics. "A bloodless diet should prove beneficial in every way, scientific, sanitary, economic, ethical, and spiritual."[15] Yet despite believing that what we refer to as a vegan diet today to be ideal ethically, he could not sustain it for long, especially after he cut out beans and rice (which he tried to eat raw), not to mention his frequent periods of fasting for civil protest, which led to a perpetually starved body.

As the nineteenth century turned into the twentieth, vegetarian advocates remained a tiny group of idealists. While most of the population got their calories from starchy plant staples such as corn, rice, potatoes, and wheat, they did so out of necessity, not choice, and certainly not moral conviction. Vegetables were linked to austerity and meat to prosperity. Meanwhile, industrialization was changing the economies of scale around meat production, and the demand for meat and dairy grew. Animals that used to be raised and killed on family farms were now bred, milked, hatched, and killed at a far larger scale, often hidden away in urban slaughterhouses. In his 1906 novel *The Jungle*, the American writer Upton Sinclair portrayed the unsanitary, dangerous, and morally degrading conditions in early slaughterhouses, and the lives of the underpaid workers who toiled there to satisfy the growing demand for meat. The book caused a public outcry that helped marshal the political will for necessary labor and human health reforms, but they left animals behind.

These social shifts—both the rapid expansion of the meat industry, and the backlash against it—attracted the attention of reformers, who began to work most actively in England, the country that first experienced the Industrial Revolution. Upper-class progressives with time and resources became involved in issues such as child labor and poverty, and they took up the animal protection cause as well. But most of their attention was focused on "companion" animals (pets) and horses, whose suffering attracted more notice than ever before. Early groups included the Royal Society for the Prevention of Cruelty to Animals (RSPCA) and the National Anti-Vivisection Society (NAVS), both of which inspired American counterparts. Still, animals raised for food consumption were largely ignored.

Alongside the moral argument for vegetarianism, this period also witnessed early stirrings for the health argument. This took form in English reformers who advocated for vegetarianism as a part of an "ascetic" lifestyle that included sleeping on hard mattresses, taking cold showers, and abstinence from sex. These early advocates believed that substances like coffee, alcohol, and meat "overstimulated" the body, and their emphasis on fasting and raw diets earned vegetarianism a reputation as spartan and bleak. Some founded movements such as transcendentalism, with one of the earliest transcendentalist communes founded in Harvard, Massachusetts, called Fruitlands. The founders (including Bronson Alcott, the father of the author of *Little Women*) went on to establish the American Vegetarian Society in New York City in 1850.

Many of these health pioneers were entrepreneurs and developed the first meat alternatives in the West. (Of course, meat alternatives have been consumed in Asia for centuries.) One was John Harvey Kellogg, a Seventh-day Adventist who created meat-like products called Nuttose (made of peanuts) and Protose (made of nuts and wheat) for patients at the Battle

Creek Sanitarium he ran in Michigan (his brother went on to establish the Kellogg's cereal brand we know today).

At first, these products were marketed to the ill, but eventually they were rebranded as "health foods" designed to optimize well-being and prevent disease. When the Sanitarium Food Company rebranded itself as Loma Linda Foods, it changed the term "meat substitute" to the more scientific-sounding "meat analogue."[16] As Dr. Kellogg wrote in 1896, "Nuts are unquestionably the vegetable analogue of meat and other animal foods, not only containing all the food elements to be found in animal products, but in finer and more digestible form, more delicately flavored, and wholly free from deleterious elements which abound in meat."[17]

Many of the early vegetarian advocates lived on the East Coast, primarily in New England. But in the mid-nineteenth century, California became an epicenter of the movement, especially as the state witnessed an influx of immigrants from the rapidly industrializing Germany. Some of those who came were part of the Lebensreform ("life reform") movement, which espoused vegetarianism, nudism, alternative clothing, and outdoor exercise. One 1917 photo shows a bearded young man in a loincloth, flanked by a house he built in the Palm Springs desert—a tableau that wouldn't have seemed out of place fifty years later during the Summer of Love.[18] Many of these "hermits," as they were called, left Germany to escape military service and became "Nature Boys," made famous by the Nat King Cole song.

These Central Europeans became pioneers of the Californian health movement, promoting a lifestyle called "natural hygiene." One notable advocate was the German immigrant Emanuel Bronner, of Dr. Bronner's Magic Soaps, famous for its preachy packaging featuring block text about health, environmentalism, and spirituality. His grandson David Bronner, Chief Empowerment Officer at the company today, continues his ancestor's legacy in more ways than one: he is a passionate vegan who supports many animal rights initiatives and promotes regenerative agriculture and the renaissance of mind-altering substances, including marijuana and psilocybin, the active ingredient in "magic mushrooms."

Another is Paul Bragg (of the apple cider vinegar brand), whose 1930s *Live Food Cookbook* promoted a vegan diet for optimal health. Bragg argued that meat was the ultimate "devitalized" food. "Bury a cow and all it does is decompose," he wrote. "Bury a peach and you can yield an orchard."[19] While some of the claims of these early advocates were not exactly scientifically rigorous, their influence cemented a link between vegetarianism and health.

Clearly, there's no linear cultural history of vegetarianism. Its roots can be traced first to Eastern religions, then to luminaries of Western thought and moralistic English reformers, and ultimately to Californian hippie health aficionados. But perhaps its starkest turn was yet to come in the cataclysm of the counterculture, when a new and far more politicized movement arose on the scene—the movement we know today as animal rights.

———

Until the 1970s, no one talked about the "rights" of animals. Then, seemingly overnight, a simple yet powerful new moral position emerged: the idea that animals are sentient beings that deserve not only moral consideration but legal rights. The idea of "animal rights" struck a chord in the postcountercultural era, since, as the sociologists James Jasper and Dorothy Nelkin write in their book *The Animal Rights Crusade*, "In the individualist culture of America, *rights talk* is often the only way to express moral values and demands. Rights—whether of patients, women, fetuses, or animals—are accepted as a moral trump card that cannot be disputed."[20]

The new animal rights organizations were completely different from those that trace their lineage back to the nineteenth century. The old guard had been interested in reform. They felt animals should be treated humanely and focused their efforts on improving welfare, while still believing in the use of animals as far as is necessary for human well-being. With their moderate tone and lack of confrontational tactics, these reformers found sympathy with the public, but they stopped short of disrupting the status quo.

The new organizations were different. Galvanized by the rhetoric of the counterculture, and inspired by the feminist and civil rights movements, they were far more moralized and confrontational than the animal protections societies that came before. They targeted scientific laboratories and cosmetic and pharmaceutical firms, fur ranchers and retailers, rodeos and circuses, hunters and trappers, slaughterhouses, butchers, even carriage drivers and zoos, with tactics that ranged from colorful public rallies to clandestine break-ins. Their language was uncompromising, and their ranks were composed of activists willing to sacrifice their time and energy—and even risk incarceration—to correct the injustices they witnessed.

The poster child for this new movement was People for the Ethical Treatment of Animals (PETA), founded by Ingrid Newkirk and Alex Pacheco in 1981. PETA was catapulted into the activist scene after pressing charges of animal abuse against a federally funded research lab in Silver Spring, Maryland. Pacheco claims to have selected the lab randomly from a list of government-funded entities and gained access to it by offering to volunteer. There he found shocking conditions: monkeys crammed in cages encrusted with feces and urine, deprived of food, and subjected to experiments in which the nerves in their limbs were severed without pain management. Pacheco brought his findings to the police, and they raided the lab, bringing animal cruelty charges against the lead researcher. The case was later overturned, since the state anti-cruelty statute did not cover federally funded research, but the researcher lost his funding.

PETA and many similar organizations were inspired by the publication in 1975 of a seminal book called *Animal Liberation*, by the Australian philosopher Peter Singer. Singer opens the book with a reminder that the idea of "animal rights" was once used to parody the case for women's rights. After Mary Wollstonecraft published *A Vindication of the Rights of Women* in 1792, the philosopher Thomas Taylor responded anonymously with *A Vindication of the Rights of Brutes*, sarcastically calling for animals such as dogs, cats, and horses to be enfranchised. Singer's point is that just as animal rights seemed absurd in the twentieth century, so too had rights for women in the eighteenth. Singer goes on to defend the unalienable rights of animals, arguing that since all sentient beings can feel pleasure and pain, they deserve equal moral regard. Echoing the utilitarian philosopher Jeremy Bentham—who stated, "The question is not, can they *reason*? Nor, can they *talk*? But can they *suffer*?"[21]—Singer writes, "If a being suffers there can be no moral justification for refusing to take that suffering into consideration."[22]

One of the enduring legacies of *Animal Liberation* is Singer's popularization of the term "speciesism," originally coined by the Oxford psychologist Richard Ryder. Singer writes, "Speciesism—the word is not an attractive one, but I can think of no better term—is a prejudice or attitude of bias in favor of the interests of members of one's own species and against those of members of other species." The concept captured the moral imagination of the animal rights crusaders who saw themselves as continuing the legacy of activists who came before them. In fact, research on the psychology of speciesism confirms not only that there is indeed a near-universal belief that humans are intrinsically more valuable than individuals of other species, but also that the tendency increases with age. This finding implies that the phenomenon is partly, perhaps even primarily, a matter of socialization, and that it could be counteracted if we were to instill different societal norms.[23]

Singer pairs his patient and logical arguments with graphic descriptions of the suffering that animals endure on factory farms and in pharmaceutical testing. This double punch left an imprint on the hearts and minds of many who became sympathetic to animals' plight and were inspired to dedicate their lives to the cause. Ingrid Newkirk writes that reading the book in 1980 was an "epiphany": "I thought, here it is, this is what I've been thinking. Someone has given a voice to it. Long after I finished reading the book, Peter Singer's words kept echoing through my mind." Before long, she gave up meat and leather and founded PETA.

An enduring legacy of the book is the popularity of the philosophy of effective altruism (known as EA) in the vegan movement, which emphasizes using evidence and reason to contribute to the greatest good. Before

Singer's book, much of the work done by animal welfare organizations was around hot-button issues like fur coats, experimentation, and circuses or zoos. While important, the fashion, science, and entertainment industries collectively impacted the lives of thousands of animals at most. Compare that to the billions—trillions, if we count aquatic creatures—who are killed in service of one industry: food.[24] Veganism became a means to an end of reducing the greatest amount of suffering among animals, and some in the movement began to consider themselves effective altruists.

While effective altruism has become controversial over recent years,[25] at the time its emphasis on rationality and impact contributed to a shift within vegan organizations. PETA and the Humane Society for the United States (HSUS) created divisions focused on farmed animals. New organizations were also established, including the Farm Animal Rights Movement (FARM), which organizes the annual Animal Rights National Conference; Farm Sanctuary; Vegan Outreach (VO); Compassion over Killing (COK); Mercy for Animals (MFA); and the Humane League (THL). While many of these organizations still promoted legislation to protect animals, there was a decisive shift toward emphasizing behavioral change in people. For the first time, veganism and animal rights merged into one movement, the chief focus of which was opposition to the relentless expansion of factory farms.

Of course, not everyone thought the movement should shift in this direction. While the animal rights tent may have seemed cohesive to outsiders, as with any movement, internal tensions began surfacing. In contrast to Singer's utilitarianism and to the welfarists who came before, some activists took a hard stance for the immediate and complete cessation of the use of animals by humans, on the grounds that animals have inherent, inviolable rights. Their philosophical position, known as "deontology," can be traced back to the work of the philosopher Immanuel Kant, but the modern animal rights philosophers advocating for this position include Tom Regan, and Gary Francione.

In *The Case for Animal Rights*, Regan points out that humans ascribe inherent value to other humans who lack rationality, such as babies and people with severe mental disabilities; similarly, since animals also have consciousness, needs, and desires, they possess inherent moral rights too, and these include the right not to be harmed. Francione, a legal scholar, combined such ideas with the notion of "abolitionism," arguing that "welfarism" (the incremental approach to improving animals' conditions) was not only counterproductive, but even destructive to the animal cause.

As with other fundamentalist groups, some of those in this movement believed that more extreme tactics were justified in pursuit of their aim of animal liberation. Perhaps the most famous group in this camp is the Animal Liberation Front (ALF), known for "direct action" such as breaking into a mink farm to release caged animals. As the "ALF Credo" proclaimed: "The ALF carries out direct action against animal abuse in the form of rescuing animals and causing financial loss to animal exploiters, usually through the damage of property. The ALF's short-term aim is to save as many animals as possible and directly disrupt the practice of animal abuse. Their long-term aim is to end all animal suffering by forcing animal abuse companies out of business."[26]

Although ALF purported to avoid violence, they did not shy away from illegal actions such as damaging property. In a famous 1984 case, members of ALF broke into the University of Pennsylvania's Head Injury Laboratory, causing $60,000 in damages and taking sixty hours of video footage that PETA later turned into the film *Unnecessary Fuss*, featuring shocking footage of researchers using machines to fracture the skulls of living primates, which led to closure of the lab.[27]

Such actions attracted swift and harsh backlash from both corporations and the state. The most consequential reaction was the Animal Enterprise Terrorism Act of 2006, which made it possible for prosecutors to charge activists not just as criminals, but as domestic terrorists. In the post-9/11 world, such activists were considered the number one domestic terrorist threat in the country, an astonishing fact given that they never actually harmed any people.

While the emphasis on ideological purity gave the animal rights movement a clear moral cause to rally around, it also alienated potential allies. Many were turned off by the movement's doggedness. The sensationalist media coverage that PETA and other organizations earned certainly spurred public debate about the treatment of animals, increased donor support, and recruited members to the cause. But radicalization ultimately cost the movement its cultural appeal. Even Singer himself advocated for a pragmatic form of activism. As he wrote, "We are more likely to persuade others to share our attitude if we temper our ideals with common sense than if we strive for the kind of purity that is more appropriate to religious dietary law than to an ethical and political movement." But many animal rights activists disagreed with this tempered attitude, and it is those with the most extreme views who captured the cultural imagination.

Despite decades of awareness campaigns, direct action, and many significant wins in reforming society, not only had the animal rights activists not met their goal of ending animal agriculture, but they had also fostered a social stigma around the term "vegan." Both literally and figuratively, the animal rights movement left a bad taste. That posed an obvious question for the activists: Where do we go from here?

Chapter Two

Paradigm Shift

The only test of rationality is not whether a person's beliefs and preferences are reasonable, but whether they are internally consistent.

—Daniel Kahneman

If I had to compare Bruce Friedrich to a fictional character, I'd choose *Star Trek*'s Commander Spock. Friedrich has a hyperlogical manner of speaking that gives you the sense he's unspooling a ready-made argument, with statistics and data never far from his tongue. "I have a very German, logic-based temperament," he admits, adding, "for better and worse." It took a lot of life experience for Fredrich to realize that, unlike him, most people do not find facts and figures nearly as convincing as stories. But that same hyperlogical nature apparently makes Friedrich immune to criticism, a quality that turned out to be a superpower for his job at People for the Ethical Treatment of Animals.

For fifteen years, Friedrich was PETA's director of campaigns. He was the mastermind behind some of the organization's most controversial campaigns against fast food chains such as KFC ("Kentucky Fried Cruelty"), Wendy's ("Wicked Wendy's"), and Burger King ("Murder King"). Friedrich believed shock tactics were necessary to wake people up to the fundamental contradiction between loving animals yet killing them for food. Once, Friedrich even streaked in front of Buckingham Palace, with "GoVeg.com" painted in green on his body, just before President George W. Bush entered the royal residence. "It worked," Friedrich told me when we first met. "We got tons of traffic to the site."

These days, Friedrich's appearance wouldn't turn heads. He's of average height and build, and he sports a clean-shaven face, crisp haircut, and square horn-rimmed glasses. He's polite and measured, and, true to his German heritage, he apologizes if he's even a couple of minutes late (which he very rarely is). But a few decades ago, Friedrich stood out in a crowd. I probably wouldn't have recognized him through the mane of long hair, the beard, and the secondhand clothes he wore. As he puts it, "I was the only one at my Catholic college who actually looked like Jesus."

Friedrich was born in 1969 in Oklahoma to a pious family. His faith has always been central to his life mission. After he graduated high school in the late 1980s, he attended Grinnell College, a small liberal arts college in the heart of Iowa. A year later, a homeless-rights activist came to give a talk and told the students that if they truly cared about the disadvantaged, they should drop out of school to help. The words sank deep into Friedrich. He felt a deep and righteous anger at the fact that his fellow Americans turned a blind eye to suffering.

After his junior year, Friedrich followed the advocate's advice and dropped out of college to run a soup kitchen in inner-city Washington, D.C., as part of the Catholic Worker movement. He was also part of the Plowshares pacifist movement, which advocated direct action in support of nuclear disarmament. In his early twenties, he and three others—a civil disobedience leader, a Jesuit priest, and a homeless-rights activist—sneaked into an Air Force base and damaged military equipment with hammers. All received felony convictions for destruction of government property, and Friedrich served fifteen months in a North Carolina prison, not the first time he had been jailed but the longest stint he'd ever served. "There's a sense among progressive Catholics that going to jail is a good thing for its own sake," he explained. "The best way to visit the imprisoned, as dictated by the Bible, is to actually be in prison." For Friedrich, it wasn't enough to give money to charity or sign a petition for the dismantling of nuclear arms. He always wanted to be on the front lines.

In fact, it was Friedrich's concern with human well-being, rather than compassion for animals, that first led him down the animal rights path. In college one of his friends suggested he read Frances Moore Lappé's *Diet for a Small Planet*, a book that, as it turned out, changed his life. Through it, he learned that raising animals for food is highly inefficient. Supplying large amounts of soy, corn, or other feed to animals yields far fewer calories in the form of meat, milk, or eggs while depleting resources such as water in the process (not to mention creating pollution). In a famous analogy, Lappé declares that a meat-centric diet is "like driving a Cadillac"— high-status, perhaps, but enormously wasteful. Reading this, Friedrich immediately became vegetarian, and shortly thereafter, vegan. "Just the idea of cycling crops through animals so we can eat them struck me as patently immoral as part of my Christian faith. It's morally equivalent of throwing that food away into the trash."

Later, a friend gave him a copy of *Christianity and the Rights of Animals* by the Reverend Dr. Andrew Linzey, an Anglican priest and professor of theology at Oxford University, which led Friedrich to realize more deeply that the plight of animals was intimately linked to his faith. Linzey makes the point that humans should, whenever possible, make kind choices rather than cruel ones. A deceptively simple message, perhaps, but a revelatory one for Friedrich: "Suddenly I saw what was happening to animals as the greatest atrocity of our time. Other animals are loved by God just as much as human beings, and yet the vast majority of people don't think about that, including Christians."

As soon as Friedrich finished the book, he told everyone he knew about what he had learned. Unlike most new vegans, he found a sympathetic audience in his parents, his girlfriend at the time, and his friends, many of whom are vegan to this day. As he later wrote, "People of integrity should choose not to support cruelty to animals, and thus should choose to eat a vegetarian diet."[1] A true Catholic, Friedrich takes the concept of not living beyond his needs very seriously. "Catholicism means that you do not live gluttonously. I don't believe anyone has the right to live conspicuously. I certainly did not want to be living my life requiring many more resources than necessary."

Learning more about animal welfare led Fredrich to leave his post at the homeless shelter and go to work for PETA in 1996. There he found a community of like-minded social justice advocates completely committed to the cause. One of them, Alka Chandra, eventually became his wife. Another, Matt Ball (cofounder of Vegan Outreach with Jack Norris), became a thought partner, and the two co-wrote *The Animal Activist's Handbook* in 2008. The book is a practical guide, teaching activists how to be as effective as possible. "Think of it this way," Friedrich and Ball write of their "vegan multiplier" strategy, which is based on leafleting in the streets: "Once we have ten people on board, our impact on the world is ten times greater than the choices that we, personally, have made *or that we will ever make*! In just *one* day, with just *one* interaction, we can do as much good for the world with our influence as we can do with our personal decisions and choices over the course of *our entire lives*."[2]

Friedrich's north star was always about being as effective as possible, and he was perpetually on the quest for the best way to raise people's consciousness about the consequences of their actions. As he wrote with Ball, "When push comes to shove, thousands of years of philosophy can be summarized in nineteen words: 'Something is "good" if it leads to more happiness, and something is "bad" if it leads to more suffering.' Because our singular goal is to have the greatest impact on the amount of suffering in the world, we've chosen to dedicate our lives to exposing the cruelties of factory farms and industrial slaughterhouses while promoting a vegetarian diet."[3]

But in 2009, around the time he turned forty, Friedrich began to have doubts about whether his efforts were truly making a difference, and he wondered about other ways he could expose people to the mistreatment of animals. Thinking perhaps that consciousness raising should begin in schools, he signed up for Teach for America. Friedrich hung MEAT IS MURDER posters in his inner-city Baltimore classroom; showed students films such as *Meet Your Meat*, narrated by Alec Baldwin, which depicts abhorrent conditions on factory farms; and had students write critical reflection pieces about the problems of animal agriculture. Friedrich hoped that if he exposed his students to animals' pain and suffering, lightbulbs would come on. But progress was slow, and Friedrich felt increasingly frustrated. He began to wonder, what does social science have to teach us about how change happens?

———

In the 1930s, a man named Everett Rogers was born on a family farm in Carroll, Iowa. As he grew up, he witnessed the first generation of American farmers who planted hybridized seed corn, and this agricultural innovation left him curious about what it takes to get people to adopt new technologies. Later, in his career as a sociologist, he theorized a "diffusion of innovations" curve that posits different "phases" in the spread of new concepts.[4] Imagine a bell curve divided into five equal sections, with each section representing a different stage in the evolution of a new technology. First come the innovators—those who, for example, bought the iPhone way before it became mainstream. Then come the early adopters, then the early majority, next the late majority, and finally, the "laggards"—people who adopt a technology only after it's widespread.

Although Rogers's theory has been mostly applied to technological developments, it can also be used as a lens to understand social movements. Historically, many social movements have succeeded in shifting the cultural zeitgeist only after decades of advocacy. It took women many centuries, and two distinct "waves" of the feminist movement, to gain the right to vote. The ongoing struggles for real equality across categories of race, sexual orientation, and gender identity also demonstrate that building mainstream consensus is long, slow work. We can even see the "diffusion of innovations" curve operating through the ebbs and flows in acceptance of mind-altering substances, including alcohol, marijuana, and, most recently, psychedelics.

For the entirety of its history, veganism has been in the "early adopters" segment of the diffusion curve—and activists like Friedrich toiled incessantly, trying to shift it into the next phase. But then something completely unexpected happened. After years of campaigning, in the early 2010s Friedrich began to hear whispers in his activist network about a new breed of vegan company emerging out of Silicon Valley. He and his friends had long been avid fans of "heritage" vegan brands like Tofurky, Gardein, and MorningStar. But as popular as these products were among vegans and vegetarians, they were ignored by everyone else. They hadn't evolved much from the early generation of meat analogues of the 1970s, made of nuts and grains, that little resembled their animal-based counterparts. The new wave of plant-based companies had a different agenda: they weren't targeting vegans or vegetarians, nor even health-conscious consumers. They wanted to appeal to the meat lover, and they were going to use "food tech" to do it.

One of the early companies in the new "alternative protein" landscape was Eat Just, known at the time as Hampton Creek. It was founded by two Joshes—Balk and Tetrick—high school friends who bonded over a love of sports and dogs. (Hampton Creek was named after Tetrick's beloved childhood pet.) After high school, both Balk and Tetrick had gone into do-good careers: Balk in the animal rights world, rising from summer intern to vice president of farm animal protection at the Humane Society of the United States, the largest and most prominent animal protection agency in the nation, while Tetrick spent time in Africa working for an education and human rights NGO. When Tetrick got back, Balk helped him to brainstorm possible career ideas and convinced him that the food industry was an ideal opportunity for real impact.

The two decided to focus on the egg industry, since chickens take the brunt of suffering among farmed animals. Broiler chickens are genetically modified so that their breasts, the part we love to eat most, are so large the birds can hardly walk. Laying hens are bound to a life of nonstop egg production, living in cages so small they are unable to turn around. Male chicks are immediately killed. Balk had worked for years at HSUS on ballot initiatives aimed at stopping such practices, with much success, but he knew that regulation would not be enough to truly change the fate of animals. They needed to work on reducing demand, too.

Drawing inspiration from the unicorn companies in vogue at the time, Uber and Airbnb among them, Balk and Tetrick decided to "disrupt" the animal agriculture industry through a signature consumer product—mayonnaise. Mayonnaise uses a lot of eggs, yet the final product is relatively easy to replicate from other ingredients. Some of their ingenuity had to do with figuring out how to make it from mung beans. But their true achievement was a keen sense of marketing. "Vegenaise" had been first to market decades prior but was selling only to vegans. Balk and Tetrick cleverly framed themselves as the underdog being bullied by the big bad egg industry, attracting not only media attention but far more capital than any previous vegan company had ever received.

In the months that followed, Friedrich witnessed companies like Eat Just, Beyond Meat, and Impossible Foods begin to gain buzz, investors' dollars, and, most important, consumers. A few of his friends asked him whether he'd consider starting a company too. Friedrich was intrigued, but he felt that his place remained that of an activist. "I really thought we just needed to educate people about the fact that there is no moral difference between eating a pet and eating a farm animal. For quite a while, I was convinced of the inevitability of our victory."

And yet despite decades of protests, demonstrations, boycotts, open rescues, and undercover footage, not to mention tons of academic papers, books, and documentaries exposing the cruelty and horror of factory farming, the consumption of meat kept rising,[5] while the number of vegetarians, much less vegans, stayed dismally low. Fredrich began thinking: "I adopted a vegan diet thirty years ago. Thirty years ago, only a tiny percent of the U.S. population was vegetarian, and that's still basically where we are now. So, while I had always thought educating people is important, I wondered if there was more we could do. We were running out of time."

Just as Friedrich began to consider the new approach taken by companies emerging from Silicon Valley, he got a call from a former intern of his at PETA. Milo (then Nathan) Runckle had gone on to start Mercy for Animals, which became one of the most influential animal welfare organizations in the country, known especially for its undercover investigations of factory farms. Runckle also noticed the Silicon Valley trend and, after talking to some of his donors, decided to fund a nonprofit to support the creation of the new plant-based industry. They were looking for a director, and Friedrich seemed like the right fit. "I told them, I'm not really into capitalism, and I don't really care about food, so I'm hardly the person to use food and capitalism to save the world."

But Runkle tried to convince him that he could create far more impact as the director of this new organization than at Farm Sanctuary, where he took a job after Teach for America. "I had lived in voluntary poverty, I had run a homeless soup kitchen for years, and I took seriously the notion that God asks of each of us to act justly and walk humbly. But he just basically wore me down. He made me see that if my goal was to make the maximum positive difference in the world, I could do a lot more at this new nonprofit."

————

At nearly the same time that some of the early Silicon Valley companies were being founded by entrepreneurial vegans, the psychologist and Nobel laureate Daniel Kahneman published the best-seller *Thinking, Fast and Slow*, based on his decades-long work with his collaborator, the late Amos Tversky. In the book, Kahneman broadly argues that humans possess two "systems" of thought. System 1 is quick, instinctual, and emotional, while System 2 is slow, deliberative, and logical. When we "go with our gut," we are operating on System 1. When we think long and hard about a problem, we are activating System 2.

The distinction between System 1 and System 2 helps to illuminate the challenge of changing our food paradigm. Our desire for calorie-dense food falls into System 1's biases, as does our preference for food that is familiar.

We gravitate toward food we grew up with and know intimately, especially if it's tied to nostalgic feelings of warmth and comfort. Our System 1 has also learned associations such as "tasty is good" and "meat is tasty," therefore "meat is good." In System 1, processing information takes almost no effort. In contrast, System 2 takes a great deal more attention and self-control. As we know, our self-control is limited, and there's only so much effort we will put into overriding the urges of our unconscious System 1.

The book was a revelation, illuminating just how irrational many of our choices can be. When Friedrich read the book, it occurred to him that our decisions around food commonly fall into the category of System 1. Most people put almost no effort into deciding what to eat, and here were the animal rights activists asking them not only to switch from System 1 to System 2, but to confront ethical dilemmas, an aspect of deliberative thinking that is especially challenging.

Behavioral science sheds light on what's known as the "meat paradox"—people consume meat *despite* knowing what goes on in the metaphoric sausage factory.[6] At play in this contradiction is the psychological phenomenon known as "cognitive dissonance," which has been observed in many domains of life. It shows that humans are motivated to rationalize behaviors that are inconsistent with our values. The psychologist Melanie Joy has shown that "three N's" are used to justify meat eating as necessary, normal, natural, and other researchers have added a fourth N—nice (that is, tasty).[7] These assumptions are baked into our System 1, and it takes significant effort to question any of those implicit associations.

Our culture, too, maintains meat eating as part of our collective psyche. A few years ago, a group of sociologists from the University of Toronto interviewed a large group of locals from all corners of the globe with a diverse set of religious backgrounds, and they found remarkable consistency in some of the tropes both meat lovers and abstainers alike used to explain meat eating.[8] They call the first set of tropes "identity repertoires," which refer to our deeply personal experiences with meat. This could be as simple as "I like the taste." People may not know why they are drawn to meat's umami flavor, which is hard to replicate with plant ingredients like tofu, tempeh, mushrooms, or nuts, but they simply feel that they can't give it up.

Men in particular draw on the identity trope "You need to eat meat to get enough protein." A thirtysomething man named Lee told the researchers, "When you look at a guy, he usually looks meatier. More flesh. So, when you see someone with more flesh, you will think, where did that person get his flesh from? Obviously from meat." In fact, the largest study comparing the nutrient intake of omnivores and plant eaters showed that the average plant eater gets not only enough protein, but far more than they need, and omnivores get half their protein from plant sources.[9] Here, System 1 is operating in full swing based on a culturally sanctioned assumption about the link between protein and muscle.

The other common identity repertoire is that of cultural preservation. Given how omnipresent meat is at family gatherings and celebrations, people worry that rejecting meat is tantamount to giving up a deep part of themselves and their community. Many respondents lamented that rejecting their grandma's turkey or another traditional communal dish would be too great a social and emotional risk. This is especially true for those for whom certain types of meat—halal or kosher, for example—are tied to their faith. In saying no to meat, they feel they are, in essence, committing a kind of religious heresy.

As the anthropologist Nick Fiddes observes in *Meat: A Natural Symbol*, meat epitomizes a complex set of cultural associations. As he explains, "It is the totality of these ideas which combine to form a language, and which constitute culture."[10] Most of the time, we're not even aware that cultural factors are at play in how we feel about something as fundamental as what we eat, and yet there they are, just beneath the surface.

Consider the young Eritrean woman called Hanna in the study, who offered, "If you were to take meat away from Eritrean culture, you wouldn't have what makes the Eritrean culture the Eritrean culture." Most cuisines around the world are based on plant-based starches,[11] with meat as merely a garnish. But in many parts of Africa, the rarity of meat situates it, for this woman as for many others, at the center of cultural belonging. She may not actively realize meat's historic association with hunting and masculinity, with group membership, and, because of its scarcity, with higher status, but she intuits that her culture would be impoverished without it.

Besides identity tropes, there are also what the researchers call "liberty repertoires," which are about more abstract notions around meat eating. One is consumer apathy, or the right to ignore inconvenient truths. Many of those interviewed framed meat eating as inevitable and attempts to fight it as naïve and disruptive. They wanted to block out unpleasant thoughts and disengage from the consequences of their choices. Sahil, an Indian meat eater in his twenties, said, "I know for a fact that meat comes from an animal, but it's just like a thought that I block or put in the back of my head." For Sahil, cognitive dissonance isn't even a coping mechanism, it's an active choice.

Finally, there's the trope of consumer sovereignty, which is about how people should have the right to eat whatever they please. Asked how he'd justify meat eating to a vegetarian, a Pakistani man named Khan in his twenties explained, "I'd say we're humans, and it's their choice if they're eating vegetables, but it's my choice if I'm eating meat, it's up to me." Some vegetarians defend meat eaters' right to choose meat, feeling they should respect their choice just as they wish meat eaters would do for them. Such a belief is especially at home in the liberal West, where personal choice, rather than moral responsibility, is of paramount importance.

No wonder animal rights activists like Bruce Friedrich failed to curb meat consumption. When Friedrich became vegan in the 1980s, he was among just 1 percent of the U.S. population. Four decades later, he's still among a tiny 3 percent. While many Americans are eating less meat, many others are eating more or simply switching from beef to chicken, which means a far greater number of animals killed (there's a lot more meat on a cow than on a chicken). Further, as people enter the middle class in industrializing nations like China and Brazil, they are drawn to the luxuries a higher standard of living affords, including meat.

After years of trying to persuade others to give up meat not only for animals, but for the planet and human health too, the activists found that only a few joined their crusade. When one argument failed, there were countless others. The activists were up against profound evolutionary drives, as well as a plethora of psychological and cultural justifications that upheld the status quo. Perhaps the most profound paradigm activists continue to confront is that of deliciousness: meat simply tastes too good to give up. Dionysus trumps Apollo.

But while the findings of behavioral science may have seemed grim for veganism, when he read Kahneman's work, it dawned on Friedrich that irrational biases could be leveraged to make better decisions easier. The approach had already been used to help people save money for retirement, choose more nutritious foods at the cafeteria, and tip more at checkout. "I realized that for most people, the choice of what to eat boils down to *How does it taste?* and *How much does it cost?*" A new theory of change was born: Don't change people, change meat. At the end of 2015, with a starting seed of $580,000 from Mercy from Animals, the Good Food Institute was born.

———

These days, the new Friedrich would probably be unrecognizable to the old. That Friedrich was a long-haired idealistic youth in baggy secondhand clothes who saw capitalism as evil and believed he could raise the moral consciousness of others by showing them the plight of the most vulnerable. The old Friedrich occasionally dumpster dived for food and drew suspicious looks from passersby and police, who followed him around in stores thinking he was about to shoplift. The old Friedrich streaked in front of the U.S. president and served a year and a half in prison for breaking into an Air Force base in an attempt to destroy a nuclear bomber with a hammer. The old Friedrich told a sociologist studying animal rights, "It will be seen as self-evident in a hundred years that eating animal corpses is no more acceptable than eating human corpses."[12]

Fast-forward a decade, and the new Friedrich wears crisp suits and horn-rimmed glasses, spends his time courting wealthy Silicon Valley investors, and invites the executives of meat companies to his conferences. In 2019, the new Friedrich told the *New York Times*, "I really thought we just needed to educate people about the fact that there is no difference between eating a pet and a farm animal, but now I know that we need to change the meat, because we aren't going to change human nature."[13]

On the surface, it seems like a 180-degree turn for this former PETA campaigner. And yet the old Friedrich is still there, just behind the veil. On the TED stage that same year, Friedrich offered a hummus and veggie sandwich to an audience member, then promptly threw eight others into the trash to demonstrate the number of calories wasted in the life cycle of a chicken. Animal agriculture supplies only 18 percent of the world's calories while taking an enormous share of plant calories in feed. For every 100 calories of crops that could be fed to humans, we get only 40 calories of milk, 22 calories of eggs, 12 calories of chicken, 10 calories of pork, and a mere 3 calories of beef![14] "Who thinks that was a good idea? No, of course not, that's a horrible idea. And yet that's essentially what meat production entails," he explained to the audience.

But while Friedrich no longer hands out leaflets or protests on the street, his ultimate mission has not changed at all. In the past, all Friedrich wanted to talk about was ethics—the ethics of eating meat while animals, the poor, and the planet suffered. He now embraces capitalism as a tool but feels it wouldn't necessarily be accurate to call himself a capitalist. "There wasn't a point at which I thought capitalism wouldn't win, I just thought it was immoral," Friedrich told me, when I pressed him on the contradiction. "But I know that what is asked of each of us is to reduce as much suffering as possible. I think that within the system of capitalism, we can do a tremendous amount of good." Yet Friedrich admits that he still doesn't understand why the vegan multiplier method doesn't seem to work. "I mean"—he paused—"it *feels* like it should work, doesn't it? But clearly it hasn't happened yet." Friedrich doesn't have time to find out if it could ever work, and neither, perhaps, do we.

Today, the Good Food Institute (GFI) lobbies on behalf of the whole alternative protein sector, surrendering the fight against all those meat-maintaining tropes the researchers discovered—especially the one about consumer apathy. But they've flipped the script and are using these tropes to their advantage. The goal is to minimize and ultimately eliminate the compromise involved in choosing between taste and ethics. Ideally, it will happen in a way that requires the least amount of effort on behalf of consumers. My guess is that if Friedrich has it his way, consumers won't even notice the change on their plates.

The "capitalist turn" embraced by vegan activists might seem radical, but in some ways it's a logical continuation of a branch of the movement that has always striven to save as many animal lives as possible. Unlike organizations like PETA, whose sensationalist tactics are about attracting media attention, these activists are in pursuit of whatever method results in the maximum reduction in suffering. That means, for some, abandoning their anti-capitalist stance and working within the system. Their mantra could easily be "The perfect is the enemy of the good."

At one of the GFI conferences, I asked Friedrich whether he still considers himself a "vegan activist," or if he tries to avoid the "v" word. He thought for a moment, choosing his words wisely: "GFI works to effectively remove animals from industrial agriculture, but the nature of our approach is not vegan advocacy. The idea of these companies is, let's create products that do not require a paradigm shift from anybody."

It turned out the paradigm shift Friedrich and his fellow activist friends were looking for didn't happen in the people they were trying to influence, but instead within themselves.

Chapter Three

Making "Meat"

Imagine what a hundred years from now will be seen as monstrous? The treatment of nonhuman animals is obvious.

—PAUL BLOOM

On a sunny morning in the summer of 2018, I hopped into a ride that took me from Venice Beach, where I was living for the summer, down to El Segundo, just south of Los Angeles and home to the headquarters of one of the emerging "it" companies in alternative protein: Beyond Meat. As the driver dropped me off in the parking lot of a nondescript building in the middle of an industrial park, I wasn't sure what to expect. On my way to the entrance, I stopped in my tracks and chuckled. Parked right out front was a red Tesla with a license plate reading BYND. At the time, the Beyond Meat headquarters were just down the street from one of Elon Musk's ventures, SpaceX. Just as Musk wants to "go beyond" our reliance on gasoline, the founder of Beyond Meat, Ethan Brown, thinks humanity can surpass our dependence on animals for the thing we crave most: meat.

I walked through the glass doors past a poster that read THE FUTURE OF PROTEIN and met the welcome staff. In typical start-up fashion, everyone was dressed as if it were casual Friday, though it was midweek. They escorted me to the CEO's office, passing by a laboratory full of beakers, microscopes, vials, pipettes, and other equipment. If I didn't know better, I'd think I had walked into the lab of a biomedical research company on a mission to cure cancer.

In a way, I wouldn't be far off. Since it was founded in 2009, Beyond Meat has been trying to cure us of the obsession we have with meat, which is ravaging our health and that of the planet. Here, scientists were analyzing thousands of molecules in beef, chicken, and pork to find those that are most like the ones in certain plants so they can extract them and recreate the taste and feel of meat in a novel way. Their ambitious goal, as Brown likes to say, is to "build meat from plants" and in so doing, if they have their way, to separate "meat" from its animal origins.

I came to the headquarters about a year before the company went public, after which Brown was suddenly surrounded by an army of public relations professionals. At the time, his office was set apart by just a glass wall on the open concept floor plan. As his meeting finished up, I was ushered in by his assistant. Brown stood up in front of his desk, flanked by four posters that reflected the pillars on which the company's mission was based— *human health, climate change, natural resources, animal welfare.* "Welcome to Beyond Meat," he said.

At least six feet tall and broad-shouldered, Brown hardly looks like what most people imagine of a vegan CEO. Brown's concern for animals and the planet can be traced to the time he spent on his family's dairy farm in Maryland. As a child, he began to feel uncomfortable with how we treat animals. When a cow was put to death on the farm after breaking a hip, he remembers thinking, "We'd never do that to our dog." As he grew older, he realized there were only degrees of difference between humans and other species: "When you put on a pair of leather shoes, you are putting on someone's mother, someone's child. It was about animal rights in the beginning, but it was also a spiritual thing, and I was concerned about the planet."

Brown thought he might become a veterinarian, but as a student at Connecticut College, he took an environmental ethics course that had a profound influence on his life path. The professor, Lawrence Vogel, taught that ethics should, above all, be pragmatic—an "antiphilosophy"—which had a deep impact on Brown.[1] Eventually, Brown got a master's degree in public policy and then an MBA from Columbia. He spent a decade in the clean energy sector but kept thinking about the food system and its outsize contribution to the environmental crisis. An avid vegan who still missed eating meat, he wondered how people could be convinced to stop eating it. He thought of his father, an environmental studies professor, who still ate meat occasionally. He asked himself, "Do we need animals to make meat?"

In search of answers, Brown mined the place that many entrepreneurs ignore: academia. Delving into the scientific literature, he happened upon the work of Fu-hung Hsieh, a professor of biological engineering and food science at the University of Missouri. What stood out to Brown was Hsieh's paper on extrusion technologies—basically a machine that can imbue soy and other legumes with chewy tissue-like texture—which came out in the *Journal of Food Science* in 2016.

Since the early 1990s, Hsieh had been studying how heat, pressure, and high moisture can transform plant-based ingredients into a fibrous material with sensory and structural similarities to meat. Hsieh's interest stemmed from his experience growing up in Taiwan, where far more people eat meat-like products made mostly of soybeans. "You need lots more land, lots more water, lots more energy to get a pound of chicken" than a legume like soy, Hsieh said.[2] With funding from the soy industry and the U.S. Department of Agriculture, Hsieh teamed up with Missouri engineer Howard Huff, and the two toiled to create a chicken-like product from soybeans.

Intrigued, Brown visited the lab, and Hsieh and Huff showed him the extruder, a machine invented in the 1870s to make sausage. In go the dry and wet ingredients and out comes a chewy fibrous material that resembles the texture of chicken. Then artificial flavorings and dyes are added that make the mixture resemble the color and taste of meat. Unlike the first generation of "meat analogues" that were dry and crumbly, Hsieh's work suggested a pathway to a better plant-based product. Brown persuaded the pair to commercialize: "They needed an entrepreneur, and I needed the scientific expertise." Brown licensed the intellectual property of the technology from the University of Missouri, set up a manufacturing facility at the university, and began raising a seed round to take the product to market.

In 2010, a year after Brown officially founded the company, the new technology was announced by the University of Missouri, and the announcement was unexpectedly picked up by *Time* magazine. Brown began to get calls from interested investors, including, to his amazement, Kleiner Perkins Caufield & Byers, calling from Palo Alto, California. Perhaps the best-known Silicon Valley venture capital firm, its star-studded portfolio includes Google, Amazon, Spotify, Peloton, EA, and Slack. This was Brown's moment, and he seized it.

On the day Brown came to Kleiner Perkins, he was interviewed by Twitter's Biz Stone, who's "veganish" (as is Stone's Twitter cofounder, Evan Williams). As Stone later told me, "I honestly thought he'd be a hippie guy and it would be another novelty food item." But Stone was blown away by the magnitude of Brown's thinking. "Ethan said he didn't want to preach to the choir. He wanted to convince carnivores that there's a perfectly good other source of delicious protein. If we do things right, we can make the same thing and scale it up and it would have a massive impact." Impressed, Stone invested through Kleiner Perkins, along with another firm, Obvious Ventures.[3] Those investments gave the new company enough clout that within a few years, they attracted a truly astonishing lineup of celebrity investors, including Leonardo DiCaprio, Snoop Dogg, and Bill Gates.[4]

What Stone found most inspiring was Brown's aim to make vegan food for nonvegans. As Seth Goldman, a former adviser to Beyond Meat, explained to me: "Our product is vegan and meets every standard a vegan would hold it to, but we are in no way trying to make this the best-selling veggie burger. If at the end of the day this becomes the most popular product among vegans and vegetarians but doesn't succeed in penetrating into the mainstream, then we will not have considered this a success. The predominant audience is much bigger, and part of that is because we are merchandising it in the meat section. If we sold it only in the fringe, then we would only get the vegans."

On the day I visited Beyond Meat's headquarters, I was led on a tour of the lab by Dariush Ajami, at the time the Chief Innovation Officer. Ajami showed me a molecular analysis comparing conventional pork sausage to texturized pea protein and the final product, Beyond Sausage. We passed by a few newly minted PhDs clad in white lab coats working, I was told, exclusively on color. I noticed several vials of plant liquid on the lab bench— cabbage, radish, carrot, paprika, tomato, and beet among them. The team was testing them to improve the look of the products. So far, beet is the clear winner.

Ajami then brought me to the room that contained the dry raw materials, where I noticed bags of soy protein, carrot fiber, and meat flavorings. These get loaded into an extruder like the one Brown first saw in Hsieh and Huff's lab. Combined with water and various plant-derived fats, the materials form the meaty texture used to create their signature products. Clearly, the whole process is a far cry from how conventional meat is produced. Early on in their endeavors, before Brown began partnering with incumbent meat companies, he was fond of remarking, "There's something wrong when you can't see how your food is made."

Ajami then led me to the lab test kitchen, where he introduced me to Marta Sajche-Menchu, Research and Development Chef. Sajche-Menchu heated up some oil and placed a couple of patties and sausages on the skillet. After a few of minutes, they were sizzling, and the Beyond Meat miracle began to unfold: Each turned, slowly, from pinkish to brown, looking and smelling like cooked meat. She placed the Beyond Burger gingerly on a bun and added the usual fixings: lettuce, tomato, onion, and mustard. Both Sajche-Menchu and Ajami watched intently as I picked up the burger, examining it from all sides before carefully taking a bite.

It tasted, predictably, quite like meat, with the chewy, fatty umami flavor and consistency of the burgers I remember eating as a child at McDonald's after volleyball practice with the team. At that point I hadn't tasted meat in a decade, so I could hardly speak to its true equivalence to conventional products, but to me, the resemblance was striking. All at once, I thought of all the people who would never dream of giving up meat, and the scope of Brown's vision came into sharp relief.

There was no denying that Beyond Meat was on to something: eating meat is about not only flavor and texture, but the whole *experience* of meat. We eat with our eyes, not just our stomachs, and there are many taken-for-granted rituals around meat consumption. We used to hunt, of course, but these days our experience typically begins in a grocery store, where we buy it raw before storing and eventually cooking it. Beyond Meat has worked to stimulate all our senses, capturing that elusive pink-to-brown hue transformation to ensure their patties don't just smell and taste like meat, but they look and *feel* like it too.

Unlike previous generations of meat analogues, which tried to be *similar* to meat, Brown envisions creating a replacement indistinguishable from the animal version. The way he sees it, current meat production involves feeding large amounts of plant matter to farmed animals in order to produce meat. What if you could just take that same plant matter and shape it into much larger quantities of plant-based meat? I wondered what the world would be like if Beyond Meat's HQ replaced the modern factory farm. As Brown told me in our interview, "We have been using animals forever as a source of protein, but the reign has been long enough. Just like we have jettisoned other technologies, I think it's high time to move on to a new era."

———

Today, plant-based products are often marketed as novel, but the truth is that meat substitutes have been around for centuries in East Asia. Tofu, made of soybean curd, and soy milk, made of soybeans and water, originated in China and Japan. Seitan, formed from wheat gluten, is also from China, while tempeh, made from fermented soybeans, has its origins in Indonesia. From their inception, tofu and tempeh were mostly seen as substitutes for meat among those who could not afford animal flesh.

A common saying in some parts of China refers to "bean milk" (soy milk) as the "poor man's milk" and bean curd (tofu) as the "poor man's meat."[5]

The first iterations of meat "analogues" in the West were made by John Harvey Kellogg at his Battle Creek Sanitarium in Michigan two hundred years ago, as well as by other Seventh-day Adventists. When textured vegetable protein (TVP) was developed in the 1960s, it became the basis of many meat substitutes that began to appear at the health food stores of the countercultural '70s, giving way to the "legacy brands" like Tofurky, Boca Burger, and Gardenburger, all founded in the '80s.

Despite their various iterations, the common thread among all these products is that they were created for (and usually by) those who identified as vegan or vegetarian for health or ethical reasons and were going out of their way to find alternatives to eating animals. But the truth is that plant-based meat "pucks," protein powders, and soy milks didn't taste like their animal counterparts. Many had an unappetizing smell and taste, and they weren't practical—originally, soy milk often came in powdered form, and you had to stir it with water to consume it like milk.

Unfortunately, the literal bad taste of many of these products left a metaphorical bad taste, and the new generation of plant-based companies have had to grapple with the enduring stereotype. The new companies—we might call them "plant-based 2.0"—are in an arms race to create products aimed not at vegans, but at meat eaters who crave the experiential, embodied, and visceral experience of the animal products they know and love. This, it turns out, is quite the technological challenge.

Not only is there the issue of flavor (meat is umami and smoky, milk is slightly sour, eggs are sulfurous) and texture (meat is chewy and dense, milk is smooth and creamy, eggs are silky and runny), but animal products are also incredibly versatile in terms of what we expect them to do. Take a moment to consider all the things we expect from eggs, for example. Depending on the dish, we might want the eggs to clump together, as in an omelet or quiche. Or we might want an egg to solidify when boiled, or act as a binder in a cake. The challenge for plant-based companies is to satisfy as many of these expectations as they can, while also competing with the artificially low (subsidized) prices of conventional animal products.

Advances in molecular biology and biochemistry have allowed new plant-based pioneers to "disassemble" animal products into constituent components—proteins, carbohydrates, lipids (fats), amino acids, and salt—and study how they interact to make up what we think of as "meat," "dairy," or "eggs." The gold mine for these founders is "biomimicry," which is the idea that their products be entirely indistinguishable from their original counterparts. Companies live and die based on how their product "performs" compared to the conventional ones they're trying to replace, not just in one form or in one recipe, but ideally across applications.

On tours I took of the facilities of many plant-based companies, including Beyond Meat, Impossible Foods, and Eat Just, among others, I found that the exact recipe for every product is, like the formula for Coca-Cola, a secret highly guarded by companies trying to protect their intellectual property. But the basics aren't all that hard to decipher, mostly because these plant-based products are made like most of the other foods you buy at the grocery store. The first step is the ingredients. In animal-based food, those are the flesh or by-products, whether meat, dairy, or eggs. In plant-based food, the primary ingredient is most often some kind of dry protein isolate, extracted from a whole food. The most popular candidates are the usual suspects of soy, corn, or wheat, and more recently pea, lentil, mung, rice, or chickpea.

I saw the protein extraction process for myself at the headquarters of Eat Just in the Mission District of San Francisco. That day, I joined a tour group of European egg executives who were curious to learn about the signature Eat Just Egg product. The yellow liquid resembling blended eggs can be made into a scramble and used in baked goods. A young food scientist led us around. "Look here," he said, pointing to a machine that looked like a giant 3-D printer. "That's a protein extractor. We put the food in there—rice or mung beans, for example—and out comes the protein." In the process, the whole food is stripped of its original fiber, and what's left is a kind of powder that you might see added to protein shakes.

Beyond Meat's rival Impossible Foods, founded by a former Stanford biochemist named Patrick Brown (no relation to Ethan Brown), started out using wheat for its products, just like the original vegan companies, but when the gluten-free craze proved to be a trend rather than a fad, they switched to soy. Balking the trend against GMOs, they opted for genetically modified soy grown in the United States rather than importing organic soy grown elsewhere, which would add significant climate costs in the transportation process (in other words, they prioritized environmental impact).

Beyond Meat started out with soy for its chicken product but, unlike Impossible Foods, quickly moved away from it due to the public's concerns around soy's phytoestrogens and GMOs (though misguided). They chose peas mostly because they were a relatively cheap commodity crop. As Ethan Brown has remarked consistently, "The greatest thing about peas is they're not soy."[6] Peas are also naturally gluten-free and cheap, a double win, and versatile enough that they can be transformed into the many types of products the company is trying to emulate.

U.S. peas are grown mostly in North Dakota and Montana, which have colder climates than the soybean states of Iowa, Illinois, Indiana, and Ohio. Early on, Beyond Meat made a deal with PURIS, a Minneapolis pea protein supplier. But as peas became the new "it" ingredient, the company felt pressure to "lock up" its pea supply. It turned to the French ingredient specialist Roquette Frères. In 2020, the two companies announced a three-year partnership in which Roquette planned to expand its French pea protein facility and build another—the world's largest—in Manitoba, Canada, where conditions for peas are optimal. The announcement was made shortly after Cargill, the American meat company, announced its own investment in PURIS, a clear signal that the tide was changing.

Plant-based companies often claim that their advantage, in theory, is that they have the entire vegetable kingdom at their fingertips to mine for proteins that are as close as possible to the animal ones they are trying to replicate. But in practice, less common ingredients are challenging to source, so they end up turning to well-established commodity crops of soy, corn, wheat, and now peas. Hopefully, the rising popularity of meat alternatives will lead to a revolution in a more diversified crop system, and other legumes may experience a renaissance.[7]

Just as in the recipe for a cake, after the dry raw ingredients are combined, next come the wet ingredients in the form of liquid vegetable fats. Beyond Meat and Eat Just rely on coconut oil, while Impossible Foods uses sunflower oil. The latest version of the Beyond Burger (our meat now comes in generations, like the iPhone) also contains cocoa butter, which looks like globules of fat, giving the patty a "marbled" appearance.[8] Holding it all together are various binding agents common in processed foods: gellan gum and methylcellulose for thickening, and sunflower lecithin for emulsification.

Impossible Foods is famous (or infamous, depending on your point of view) for bioengineering a novel ingredient called "heme." Heme is an iron-carrying molecule in hemoglobin which gives blood its distinct red color, as well as a slightly metallic taste. Patrick Brown began testing heme in multiple plant sources back when he worked as a biochemist at Stanford University. He found that soy leghemoglobin (that is, heme-carrying plant protein) performed the best, and eventually figured out how to manufacture it in yeast tanks.

When Impossible first debuted their heme product, they got into hot water with, of all possible critics, PETA. The animal rights organization was incensed that the company had tested its heme on rats to get FDA approval. Brown felt personally affronted by the attack. The way he saw it, it was a question of means versus ends. They experimented on a total of 188 rats with the goal of eventually avoiding the deaths of billions of cows (at least, hypothetically). "With a lot of fundamentalist religious groups," Brown told *The New Yorker*, "it's bad if you're a nonbeliever. But if you're a *heretic*— that's a capital crime."

Regardless of the base ingredients, the finishing touch is always flavoring. Peas have a strong and distinct flavor, especially in their isolate form, so it must be masked in production. Impossible Foods privileges taste above all else, using artificial flavorings to mask their protein isolate, while Beyond Meat relies on more "natural" ingredients, including beet and pomegranate extracts that give the patties the appearance of raw pink meat. Their most ingenious color-inducing ingredient is probably apple extract, which helps the patty, like a sliced apple left too long on the counter, to turn brown, which was what impressed me most when I visited their headquarters.[9]

In recent years, plant-based products have been widely criticized as "artificial" and "processed." Marion Nestle, the well-respected nutritionist at New York University and author of the book *Food Politics*, writes on her influential blog, "One of my personal rules is never eat anything artificial. These products are off my dietary radar."[10] Her concerns—echoing the voices of many other critics—are that many plant-based products contain the same old additives of the fast-food playbook—preservatives, emulsifiers, flavorings, humectants, colorants, and chemical sweeteners.[11]

No doubt, some plant-based products don't deserve the "health halo" often attributed to them. A plate of rice and beans is certainly better for you than a Beyond Burger. Then again, it's worth considering that there is a spectrum of healthfulness among plant-based products. It's also worth remembering what we're comparing these products to in the first place. In the context of Big Food, plant-based companies are no different from any other manufacturer that produces cereal, bread, cookies, jams, pasta, chocolate, and ice cream, all of which are "processed" in some way to ensure shelf stability. That's true for virtually every packaged food you'd find in the grocery store.

It's also worth noting that when meat proponents say that it is "just one ingredient," they are obscuring a darker truth. Most of the animal products consumed around the world come from industrial farms, where the feed contains fertilizer residue and antibiotics, and traces of these chemicals remain in the animals' flesh. After slaughter, meat is marinated in sodium phosphate (to retain freshness) and colored with carmine, extracted from insects, to make it appear freshly slaughtered.[12] Some meat is also treated with modified food starch, soy protein isolate, carrageenan, gums, seasonings, and flavorings to cover up the taste of decay. That's not even to mention the health concerns around animal protein itself, whether grass-fed or organic, which I'll delve into later.

Surely, you'd do best to avoid processed food altogether and eat fresh, whole, unprocessed foods. But the reality is that meat is an omnipresent part of most Americans' lives, and research has shown that when consumers purchase alternatives, they typically choose analogues that closely resemble the taste, texture, and appearance of conventional meat rather than bean or "veggie" burgers. That means the Beyond Burger goes a long way toward satisfying people's cravings.[13] Ideally, plant-based food companies would create cleaner label products with fewer and more transparent ingredients and would pay far greater attention to how their base ingredients are cultivated, and such products would be "transition" or "treat" foods, but my view is that they are certainly better than the status quo. Barbecue with a side of hormones, antibiotics, ammonia, feces, carcinogenic compounds, and insect dye, anyone?

———

One prominent founder in the vegan movement has been especially forward-thinking in terms of creating products that are truly better for animals, the planet, and human health. Miyoko Schinner of Miyoko's Creamery (she has since left the company) is not only a serial entrepreneur who built two vegan businesses long before plant-based was mainstream, but she also founded a sanctuary for animals recovering from factory farms. Her many accolades include winning a California lawsuit that gives her and others the right to call plant-based products "cheese" and "butter." As if that weren't enough, Schinner literally embodies the vegan lifestyle with "Incredibly Vegan" tattooed on her right arm.

When I toured the Santa Rosa headquarters back when she was still CEO, I was impressed by the care and craftsmanship that goes into every product they make. Inspired by traditions of French and Italian cuisine and her own experience as a chef, Schinner wanted to make delicious foods that stand on their own, unlike many of the more "processed" vegan goods created to look and taste exactly like those made from animals.

Schinner was a pioneer in applying time-honored techniques to the art of vegan cheese. Traditional cheese is made when lactic acid culture is added into milk and combined with an enzyme that eats the sugar in the mammalian fluid. This lowers the milk's acidity, coagulating it into curds. Normally, these curds are separated from the liquid and then pressed into cheese. The same basic process, it turns out, can be used for milk and cheese made from plant substrates like cashews (which are neutral in taste and high in fat but lower in protein) or other nuts and seeds such as macadamias, pumpkin seeds, or almonds, and of course soybeans. While plant milks have been around for millennia, the process of making cheese from nuts, seeds, and legumes, and especially commercializing these products at scale, is a whole new endeavor.

Schinner's standards are high, and that has brought challenges in an industry that incentivizes cheap products devoid of nutrition. In 2021, Schinner brought in a consultant to help her brainstorm new product lines. She was told to make shredded cheese people could put on pizza. But conventional cheese products are mostly oil and starch, and the plant-based product they created proved no different, even with the extra plant proteins her team added to improve nutritional quality. Schinner was never satisfied with the product, and a few months later, she pulled it off the shelves, not due to poor sales, but because she deemed it "dumbed down" and not representative of the Miyoko's Creamery philosophy. Announcing her decision, she wrote:

> I'm sorry if I disappoint, but my company is not "food tech." We are not "alt protein." We make food—simply put, we are the natural evolution of cheese making from animal milk to plant milk . . . It is not "technology" or the "product" that is going to save this planet or mankind, but the spirit with which we create what we create.[14]

I asked Schinner to describe her vision of how we could eat in the future, and she emphasized the importance of keeping the big picture in mind. "I think it's important to have a holistic viewpoint of the food system. We should be asking ourselves, how is what we're making going to impact animals? How will it impact the planet? How will it impact people—their wages and their ways of life? Will the system be democratized or is it going to further consolidate our food sector? If we're still going to have the inequities that we have today, are we going to be adding to the problem?"

No doubt, in the last decade, founders like Ethan Brown and Miyoko Schinner have changed the game by widening the market beyond tried-and-true vegans. Yet despite the meteoric rise of plant-based products, it's still unclear whether they will truly convince die-hard meat and dairy lovers to switch. Whatever the founders may claim, peas and soy aren't, at the end of the day, meat, and many consumers still complain about not being able to find a cashew-based cheese that satisfies their cravings. Maybe what we need in order to replace these products are meat and cheese made in entirely new ways.

Chapter Four

Meat without Misery

Animals are the main victims of history, and the treatment of domesticated animals in industrial farms is perhaps the worst crime in history.

—Yuval Noah Harari

It's a crisp December day in San Francisco, and my husband, Douglas, and I have crossed the Bay Bridge from Oakland to meet with Dalton Thomas. Thomas is a former chef who now leads tastings at Wildtype, a start-up that raised $100 million in its Series B round (their investors include Leonardo DiCaprio, Jeff Bezos, and a whole roster of professional athletes)—the largest sum ever for a company making what they call "cultivated" seafood. In the span of just a few months, they have more than doubled in size and are expanding their pilot facility to support the commercial launch of their signature product: raw sushi, grown from animal cells in a laboratory.

The product has not yet been cleared by the Food and Drug Administration, but Wildtype is working on clearing the regulatory hurdles. In the meantime, they showcase their signature product at "the Dock," a tasting room at their headquarters. Wildtype HQ is located in San Francisco's

Dogpatch neighborhood, today the site of the many biotechnology start-ups. Walking down the hallway, we passed by several "boho industrial" offices: large open rooms with high warehouse ceilings decorated with charming potted plants and midcentury furniture. Thomas greeted us at the door, and Aryé Elfenbein—one of the cofounders whom I met back in 2018 at the Good Food Institute conference—gave us a welcoming hug before rejoining an adjacent meeting.

Thomas led us first to the upstairs lab unit. We passed through a room full of lab benches, whirling machines, and beakers full of reddish liquid swirling around in flasks. Then we paused outside a room in which, Thomas explained, food scientists were busy testing "cell lines" for salmon, as well as other species of fish. Cell lines can be developed directly from a living organism, with a single cell stimulated to allow it to expand into multiple cells (though no actual cloning is used). But they can also originate from a living organism and be maintained for many years, the approach used for commercially available cell lines, and the method used by Wildtype. They take a biopsy of a juvenile fish, turn those cells into stem cells, and then grow them in a bioreactor, a pressure-controlled steel vat containing a nutrient-rich broth (a "medium") that allows the cells to proliferate. The result is a mass of cells that can then be placed onto "scaffolding" (a structure on which it can grow), which allows it to scale. Essentially, the process is a kind of structural engineering at the microscopic level.

The best analogy might be how bread is made from a sourdough starter, except instead of feeding yeast sugar to convert to alcohol, the medium contains a mix of nutrients—water, glucose, salts, amino acids, hormones, proteins, and other substances that regulate cell development and metabolism—a kind of "supercharged Gatorade," as Thomas memorably described it. In theory, once the sample is taken, the cells can be grown in perpetuity, as long as they are kept in optimal temperature, oxygen, and sanitary conditions.

Thomas held out the final product, cultivated salmon saku, a plastic-wrapped block resembling the upper loin of a raw salmon fillet. It looked remarkably like a piece of salmon, with fatty sections of orange-pink flesh separated by a thin white line. Thomas explained that the masses of cells come out of the industrial tanks as an amorphous mound on three different scaffolds and the block has to be molded by hand. "As you can imagine, it's a labor- and time-intensive process, so we are exploring ways we can scale it. Right now, the business model is compatible with high-tier restaurants but not the public just yet."

The cost of cell-cultured meat is still prohibitive, and many are skeptical that it will ever reach parity with conventional meat. Wildtype's two competitor companies—Finless Foods in Berkeley and BlueNalu in San Diego—also focus on fish species with exceptionally high price points ($100 per pound) and endangered status. When Wildtype first debuted its product back in 2020, it cost about $200,000 per pound to produce.[1] Nowadays an eight-piece sushi plate is $40—still expensive, but certainly feasible for the high-end sushi market. Entering high-end markets first follows the precedent set by other technological industries. Consider Tesla, which offered the Roadster and Model S to wealthy consumers before the mass-produced Model 3.

I wondered what they would call the product when they began to market it more widely. So far, their focus group research has shown "cultured salmon" to be the preferred term, but how to accurately describe the ingredients on labels? The first and dominant ingredient, as with natural salmon, is water. But the second is real salmon, made of salmon cells. Although accurate, "salmon cells" doesn't exactly sound appetizing on the back of a package. Many of the leaders in this space are concerned about the controversy and subsequent consumer pushback around genetically modified organisms (GMOs), so proper labeling is a critical hurdle.

We came back out of the lab and waited in the welcome area while their chef prepared a platter of coho salmon sushi rolls for our tasting. He handed Thomas a plate resembling a shell—Wildtype's branding is on point. There were eight rolls, complete with all the normal fixings—soy sauce, white rice, and wasabi—and, right on top of each, a thin slice of "salmon" looking very much the part of raw sashimi. The presentation was certainly convincing, but of course, it would all be for naught without the key ingredient: taste.

———

Thomas led us downstairs to the Dock. As we stepped outside, a crisp ocean breeze wafted our way, reminding us of the bigger picture behind their whole enterprise. Global seafood production has quadrupled since the 1970s.[2] As consumers turned away from red meat, they began eating far more wild-caught fish, leading to fish stocks becoming overexploited.[3] Aquaculture—or "fish farming"—was originally intended as a solution to this problem, but instead, consumers simply continued to eat more fish. This trend led to fish farming growing sixfold since 1990, while the rate of wild-caught fish consumption has stayed at the same critical level.[4] Overall,[5] less than 3 percent of the world's oceans are "protected" from fishing.[6]

A large industrial garage door began to open, revealing what looked like a poke bar by the sea. To our right was a beach bar complete with wooden canopy, plants, and hanging lights. The walls, painted with big blue waves, proclaimed inspiring catchphrases: THE FUTURE OF SEAFOOD, THERE'S A WILD WORLD OUT THERE, WAITING FOR YOU, and the company's raison d'être: ON A MISSION TO CREATE THE CLEANEST, MOST SUSTAINABLE SEAFOOD ON EARTH. The overall effect was that of a tastefully designed, boho chic, social-media-friendly restaurant.

Behind it stood tall glass doors revealing their pilot facility. It looked like a brewery, full of steel tanks and other industrial equipment. In fact, the analogy is one embraced by the cell-cultured meat industry as a whole. Not only is it a familiar concept, but it helps to create the sense of transparency—the opposite of any conventional meat producer. Will people one day take tours to see where their meat comes from, I wondered? Clearly, that's the impression Wildtype intended to make.

Thomas took his place behind the bar, setting the plate down between blue Japanese-style dishes, and Douglas and I took our seats. Slowly, I placed the whole roll on my tongue, the "raw" flesh touching the top of my mouth.

The flavor was unexpectedly mild, much less "fishy" than I recall fish tasting. The texture, too, was different: creamy, and far softer and squishier. Granted, it had been years since I tasted raw sushi, so I was curious what Douglas thought. He had eaten more sushi in his life, and more recently, which is why I brought him along. He smiled widely. "Wow, this truly is wild."

"The smell is far less intense than I remember of conventional salmon," I remarked. "Can you tell us why?" Thomas explained that in fact, freshly caught salmon actually has quite a mild flavor. It's only when it's left out, and the fats are exposed to oxygen, that resident bacteria slowly advance, creating a "fishier" smell. How strange, I thought, that the umami flavor we crave in seafood might actually be the flavor of bacteria, kind of like a smelly cheese.

I had to admit that the texture, too, needed work. I picked the salmon up off the top of my next roll and examined its consistency. It didn't have the fibrous texture of conventionally raised salmon. It was too soft and pillowy to look like muscle. Thomas explained that in some ways, the product is too "perfect"—in nature, salmon flesh grows, moves, and even tears, creating tissue scars and other irregularities that we associate with the texture of meat and fish. The company is applying methods from the textile industry, spinning wet fibers to help give the flesh an "irregular" quality that appears authentic. Who knew that innovations in food could be inspired by the textile industry?

Right now, Wildtype's signature product is raw sashimi, but they are exploring other types of fish. Perhaps surprisingly, the salmon they've crafted is not easily cooked. It can be torched, but unlike a natural piece of meat, which has grown within the context of a body, the mass of cells that make up cultivated meat doesn't know how to "behave" like meat, and while it can be consumed raw, it can't be baked, fried, roasted, or blowtorched, as it will disintegrate. Cell-cultured companies are facing the same challenge as plant-based ones: the versatility of animal products and the challenge of replicating not only the taste and texture, but also the "performance" we expect from each.

Wildtype has managed to impress its most important advocates—chefs—many of whom no longer want to serve salmon due to concerns around overfishing and sustainability. It's also an optimal solution for consumers, since wild-caught salmon, even for all its health benefits, is fished from polluted waters containing microplastics, parasites, and mercury. (It's worth mentioning that fish get their DHA, a type of omega-3, by consuming algae, so it's possible to get the same healthful fats from seaweed directly, as well as from walnuts, flaxseeds, and chia seeds.)[7] Wildtype has been running lab tests to compare their product to conventional (both wild-caught and farmed) salmon for years, and every piece of conventional fish they tested contained some level of mercury, while even pregnant women can eat Wildtype's fish.

There was no doubt that the product was a more convincing replica of flesh than some of the plant-based alternatives I've tried that were made from components like carrots and tomatoes, but it still had a long way to go. As with any other technology, though, there will be successive iterations, and I found the product impressive for its stage. I could see why they managed to attract impressive amounts of capital and investor interest. As we left the Dock that day, there was no doubt in my mind that should Wildtype and the other companies in this space succeed, we are standing on a precipice of an entirely new food system such as we have never known before.

———

Wildtype's origin story goes back to the autumn of 2011, when Aryé Elfenbein was deep in his cardiology internship at Yale School of Medicine, working hundred-hour weeks. He barely had time to feed himself, much less cook for anyone else. But one day, he got an invitation that piqued his curiosity: a dinner at which everyone invited knew no one besides the host. The idea was to spark unexpected connections. Elfenbein decided to attend, despite the stress of having to make something for the occasion. His "I don't have time to cook" cranberry crisp in hand, he went—a decision that turned out to be a pivot point in his life.

That evening he happened to sit next to Justin Kolbeck, who had just returned from Pakistan on an assignment for the Foreign Service. Working seven days a week from a military base in the midst of a war zone, Kolbeck witnessed the extremes of poverty, putting his own modest background as the eldest of six children raised on food stamps into sharp global relief. The experience was traumatizing in many ways, and he was still recovering from a bout of tuberculosis. Intending to stay in the Foreign Service, Kolbeck convinced the State Department to pay for part of an MBA at Yale, a program known for its mission-driven culture.

Elfenbein, too, cared about making an impact. Before residency (he holds both an MD in cardiology and PhD in vascular biology), he did postdoctoral work in Kyoto, Japan, where he worked at the lab that made the Nobel Prize–winning discovery that stem cells could be made from ordinary skin cells rather than embryos. Prior to this momentous insight, there was a moratorium on stem cell research in the U.S. due to ethical issues. Suddenly, whole new avenues of possibility opened in "regenerative medicine," a field focused on developing tissues and organs and restoring functionality after tissue damage, disease, or aging.

Despite the vast differences in their professional backgrounds, Elfenbein and Kolbeck bonded instantly over their shared desire to create a better world. The two bonded even more deeply when Kolbeck helped Elfenbein recover after he was assaulted on the streets of New Haven, suffering a jaw fracture, a black eye, and two missing front teeth. "Justin took care of me in a way I'll never forget," said Elfenbein, visibly moved even years later. "He came over to make me shakes to drink—he was very concerned that I wouldn't get enough protein—so it was a friendship first."

The pair spent many weekend mornings talking over coffee, sometimes spitballing ideas for companies they might start together. Many were questionable—one was for a new kind of neti pot. But others held more sway over their imaginations, such as the one inspired by Elfenbein's trip back home to Australia during graduate school.

Visiting his family in the northern part of the country, Elfenbein noticed that much of the forest he remembered growing up around had been cleared for grazing cattle. He remembers a funny thought popping into his mind, coincidentally the same one that entered Ethan Brown's head a few years earlier: *Do we need animals to grow meat?* But for Elfenbein, with his background in stem cell research, that idea led to an entirely different conclusion: real meat grown directly from animal cells, no slaughter involved.

For Kolbeck, who had seen firsthand how food scarcity can ravage a population, the idea of culturing meat "plugged into a massive societal hole." He was always thinking about how to make nutritious food as cheaply and abundantly as possible, and culturing meat seemed like an efficient way to do it. "Why raise and slaughter animals when you could use basic raw materials like amino acids, salts, and sugars to create meat?" No wasted time, resources, and energy to grow bones, hooves, horns, vital organs, and muscles.

The idea, as much as it might sound like science fiction, has been around for at least a century. As far back as 1931, Winston Churchill made the often-quoted statement: "We shall escape the absurdity of growing a whole chicken in order to eat the breast or wing, by growing these parts separately under a suitable medium."[8] That's exactly what various labs tried to do throughout the twentieth century, with NASA even attempting to grow "space meat" for astronauts before abandoning the project.[9]

But it was not until the early 2010s that the concept was developed. In 2011, Mark Post, a scientist at Maastricht University in the Netherlands, told the *New Yorker* that cultured meat technology was possible but simply lacked enough funding. Within weeks, an anonymous donor—later revealed to be Google cofounder Sergey Brin, a longtime vegetarian—gave them $330,000 to get started.[10] In 2013, Post debuted the first "cultured" burger at a landmark press conference in London. Although the five-ounce patty cost $300,000 to produce, and reportedly hardly tasted like actual meat, it nevertheless signaled that the slaughter-free burger could one day become reality. To ethical and environmental vegans, it was a beacon of hope, inspiring many with a bold new vision of what the future of food could be.

In a twist of fate, Elfenbein had actually worked in the same lab as Mark Post, years before he met Kolbeck. "I thought 'Oh look, now Mark's making burgers.'" He decided to attend the First International Symposium on Cultured Meat, hosted by Maastricht University in collaboration with New Harvest, a nonprofit research institute that has been instrumental in developing cell-cultured meat technology and coined the term "cellular agriculture" to describe the space.[11]

With only thirty participants, the conference represented the pioneering days of cultured meat. Many of the industry's key figures were in attendance, including Isha Datar, the executive director of New Harvest. A molecular biologist by training, Datar had just published a landmark paper on what was known as "in-vitro meat."[12] Ever since, she has been instrumental in lining up financial and scientific support for many founders. She helped found Perfect Day (originally Muufri) and the EVERY Company (originally Clara Foods), which are technically "acellular agriculture" companies since they use techniques such as biomass or precision fermentation. Fermentation has been used for millennia to create products as diverse as beer, miso, and sauerkraut, and recently biotech companies realized the technology could be used for alternative proteins as well.

Precision fermentation involves the use of microbial hosts as "cell factories" for functional ingredients, including enzymes, flavoring agents, proteins, vitamins, fats, and natural pigments, and can be used to bioengineer key ingredients that we used to source from animals. Already, much of the cheese you eat today has been made with bioengineered rennet (curdled milk) that used to be taken from the stomachs of ruminant animals. Insulin, too, used to be harvested from the pancreas of slaughtered pigs, but it is now synthesized with yeast. Not only are the lab versions less cruel, but they are also more hygienic. Biotech companies began working on deriving ingredients like gelatin and collagen (Geltor), dairy (Perfect Day), and egg whites (EVERY) for sale to other companies.

There was a special energy at that original symposium. Elfenbein attended purely "as a voyeur," he thought, but by the end of the event his mind was spinning. Seemingly overnight, a whole new industry was born, and a technology that had long been confined to academic laboratories suddenly represented an opportunity for aspiring entrepreneurs—and investors. Cellular agriculture had entered its "start-up" phase.[13] In the years that followed, the number of companies in the space grew precipitously. When I began doing research on the topic as a graduate student in 2017, there were only a handful of companies globally, but by the time I defended my dissertation in 2020, there were dozens.

Mark Post went on to start his own company, called Mosa Meat, in the Netherlands, but the epicenter of the innovation was once again Silicon Valley, and a handful in the "start-up nation" of Israel. One of the earliest was Memphis Meats (later renamed Upside Foods), cofounded by Nicolas Genovese (who had attended the symposium) and Uma Valeti. In an interview with the philosopher Sam Harris for an episode of the popular *Making Sense* podcast (called "Meat Without Misery," from which I borrowed this chapter title), Valeti vividly recalls witnessing the slaughter of chicken and goats at a birthday party in India: "There was a birthday and then there was a death day, all in the same span of time, and it disturbed me. But I liked the taste of meat and I continued to eat it."[14]

Many years later, Valeti witnessed Mark Post's debut of the cultured burger and was inspired by the potential of cultured meat technology. Valeti was an established cardiologist at the world-famous Mayo Clinic, and he wasn't looking for a career change. But one day, using novel stem cell technology to repair cells after a cardiac arrest, it dawned on him: *If stem cells can be cultivated to replace heart muscle, why can't they be grown into a piece of meat?*[15] When he saw Post's debut, he was inspired to start a company of his own. Within a few years, Upside Foods (originally Memphis Meats) produced a cultured meatball, followed by both chicken and duck meats. By 2020, Upside Foods secured a landmark $161 million in their Series B round of funding.

But no one yet was working on fish. Until, that is, Elfenbein and Kolbeck began brainstorming about how to fill the gap. Inspired by Elfenbein's trip back home to Australia and Kolbeck's work abroad, they joined heads around creating a cultivated meat product. By that time, Elfenbein had moved to San Francisco to take a position as a critical care cardiologist and molecular biologist at the Gladstone Institutes, a state-of-the-art biomedical research institution, and Kolbeck had left the Foreign Service and settled in Seattle but continued commuting to the Bay Area for his consulting job. They decided to invest their hard-earned savings to rent a lab by the hour on nights and weekends.

Elfenbein had the scientific expertise, and Kolbeck the business background, but it turned out Kolbeck was a natural scientist too. Elfenbein taught Kolbeck how to isolate cells, maintain sterile conditions, and identify when and how to adjust parameters for optimal growth—"I've never seen somebody show up and just get so good at cell culture so quickly," Elfenbein said admiringly of his cofounder. The pair learned a lot about how cells behave, including how they take on different "careers"—as skin, fat, and muscle cells.

Their quest was to induce cells to take on different careers not through a natural process, but from the plant-based scaffolds provided in the lab. Through experimentation, they found that harder plant cells cued animals cells to become proteins, while softer plant cells cued animal cells to turn into fat. At first they experimented with chicken and duck cells, since it proved difficult to get access to the kinds of endangered fish species they were most interested in working on. While both still held down demanding full-time jobs, coming to the lab felt like fun, not work. "Our friends were going out for drinks, and we were coming to our lab bench to do experiments. It was the kind of enthusiasm I felt in college, where every moment was a sense of discovery. I think that was the spark."

Eventually, the cofounders felt that they had made enough progress on cell lines and plant-based media formulations that leaving their day jobs seemed like a realistic prospect. Elfenbein chose to continue being a critical care cardiologist once a week, but Kolbeck left his consulting job entirely to work on pitch decks and take meetings with potential venture capital investors. Luckily, the timing was just right. With the initial seed funding—$3.8 million in 2018—they were able to hire a small team, courting talent away from established companies like Genentech with the promise of a potentially world-shifting scientific adventure.

Their mission from the beginning was to replicate nature as closely as possible, even down to the name they chose for their company. "Wildtype" is defined as the phenotypical form of a species. Essentially, its ideal form. "It's an homage to the perfection of nature," explained Kolbeck. "We'll never one hundred percent replicate exactly what nature is doing, but to us it's a call to action." Perhaps, if they succeed, one day our own grandchildren will be shocked that we used to slaughter animals for meat rather than simply cultivating them the way we brew beer.

———

Despite the excitement around the cell-cultured meat industry on the part of investors, future consumers, and prominent journalists like Ezra Klein, who published a piece called "Let's Launch a Moonshot for Meatless Meat" in the *New York Times*,[16] there are still many unanswered questions. Skeptics are concerned about the price, arguing that current iterations of meat require enormous resources to produce, and especially with the government subsidies reducing the cost of conventional meat, cell-cultured meat will never reach price parity. One prominent analysis showed just how difficult it would be.[17] As an expert commented in a blockbuster piece for *The Counter*, "It's a fractal no. You see the big no, but every big no is made up of a hundred little nos."[18]

In 2021, Eat Just set world records by serving the first cultured meat burger at a restaurant in Singapore.[19] At $23, it wasn't cheap, but it was a bargain compared to Mark Post's burger unveiled a few years before. Still, it's hard to imagine it ever being as cheap as a conventionally grown and slaughtered chicken nugget.

Apart from cost, naysayers point to the technical challenges. When I visited the Alt Meats Lab at UC Berkeley, its director, Ricardo San Martin, a tissue engineer, expressed skepticism that cultured meat would be feasible at scale. The problem, he said, is that cells simply don't behave the same

way on the lab bench as they do in large bioreactors, and there are biological constraints on how many cells can multiply in confined conditions. He
explained that when muscle cells grow too thick, oxygen and nutrients
cannot penetrate as effectively, and cells begin to die. They also require
fastidious sterilization practices to prevent contamination. Since they don't
have immune systems to protect them, they are vulnerable to viruses.[20]

Other skeptics are concerned about the ethics surrounding the medium,
or nutritious fluid, in which cells are grown. In the early days, companies
primarily relied on fetal bovine serum (FBS)—blood drawn from a cow's
fetus. While its use is widespread in the biotech world (especially in stem
cell research) due to its growth properties, cell-cultured meat companies
can't exactly claim to be "slaughter-free" if they use this growth medium.
Companies (including Wildtype) have reportedly developed their own
plant-based mediums using conventional ingredients (my guess is the usual
soy), but it's not yet clear whether they can scale either, or whether other
technical challenges will arise.

Still others worry about the general safety and transparency of the technology. The debate around Monsanto and genetically modified food rages
on, giving biotech a bad reputation in the food world. Although cell-
cultured meat companies use unmodified cells, technically considered
non-GMO, I still envision backlash if the technology is not presented in
detail to regulators and consumers.[21] Heeding these worries, many companies, including Wildtype, have taken preemptive measures to get FDA
officials on board with their product development process. Thanks to proac-
tive engagement by the industry, the USDA and FDA reached agreement
in 2019 on the responsibilities of each agency for regulating cell-based meat.
The USDA is responsible for regulating the manufacture and labeling of
food products derived from the cells, while the FDA oversees cell collec-
tion and development of cells to harvest.

In 2022, Upside Foods was the first company to receive a letter from the
FDA stating that the agency had "no further questions" regarding the safety
of Upside's chicken product. This "green light" created reverberations for

the feasibility and acceptance of the technology worldwide. In July 2023, Dominique Crenn's Bar Crenn—a Michelin-starred restaurant that took meat off the menu in 2018—became the first restaurant in the world to serve Upside Foods' cultivated chicken.[22] Seafood is primarily regulated by the FDA, so for Wildtype, only FDA approval is needed.

Perhaps the biggest open question is whether the revolutionary meat will have a substantially smaller environmental footprint. Early life-cycle assessments (LCAs)—a method used to evaluate the environmental impact of a product—suggest that compared to conventional beef, cell-cultured would reduce greenhouse gas emissions and usage of energy and decrease the use of water by at least 75 percent and of land by a whopping 99 percent.[23] Yet newer findings show that the environmental impact of cultured meat depends substantially on medium composition and especially on whether renewable energy is used in the lab.[24,25] The predictions are speculative, so we have to wait for analyses of real products before definitive conclusions can be drawn about cultured meat's environmental footprint.[26]

Given its revolutionary potential, it's no surprise that this technology has received a lot of pushback, especially from the deep-pocketed meat industry. One of the most controversial issues has been around the nomenclature. Right now, the USDA defines meat as "any product . . . made wholly or in part from any meat or other portion of the carcass" and the FDA defines meat as "part of the muscle of any cattle, sheep, swine or goats which is skeletal," categories that don't appear to admit of the inclusion of real meat grown from animal cells.

In 2019, the National Cattlemen's Beef Association introduced legislation in the U.S. Senate called the Real MEAT (Marketing Edible Artificials Truthfully) Act. The bill attempts to restrict the use of the term "meat" (as well as "beef," which is their special interest) to refer only to products that derive from animals born, raised, and harvested in a traditional manner.[27] Since then, a handful of states have passed meat labeling laws. In response, GFI is challenging these laws on First Amendment grounds. The debate continues, with those defending the new technology preferring the terms "cultured" or "cultivated" while many ranchers and farmers who oppose the new technology prefer "synthetic," "fake," or "lab-grown."

This debate is analogous to the one spurred by another lab-grown product: diamonds. When diamonds were first synthesized, the diamond industry claimed that lab-grown diamond jewelry couldn't possibly symbolize "forever," a muddy concept at best. Lobbyists even tried to convince the Federal Trade Commission (FTC) to define the diamond as a "natural" mineral, but the FTC decided, in the end, that diamonds are diamonds, whether harvested from the earth or cultured in a lab. However, as the public became more aware of "blood diamonds," lab-grown diamonds became more popular, and the industry eventually succumbed. Many of the major brands now offer lab-grown versions for much less than the price for mined diamonds. If lab-grown meat goes the same way as diamonds, one day it may seem strange for consumers to choose "natural" meat as opposed to "lab-grown."

No doubt there are still many financial, technical, environmental, and political challenges facing the cell-cultured meat industry. But a world in which people can have their meat and eat it too, without the mass slaughter of animals and depletion of planetary resources, is a world I'd like to live in. The technology may even address one of the biggest threats of our generation: the risk of antibiotic resistance[28] and zoonotic diseases.[29] Imagine a future in which hygienically and ethically cultivated meat becomes the norm, and hunting or killing animals is the exception. Our descendants may look back at our time as the Dark Ages of agriculture. Cell-cultured meat may light the way to a new era.

Just a few weeks ago, as Douglas and I were driving home to Oakland from downtown San Francisco, I pointed out a billboard for Perfect Day's Brave Robot, an ice cream made of animal-free dairy.[30] "Wait, *animal-free dairy?* What does that even mean?" he asked.

"Basically," I explained, "they take microflora, which is like yeast, encode it with the DNA sequence for whey—that is, milk—protein, ferment it in a tank like the one we saw at Wildtype, filter out the milk protein, and engineer it to be lactose-free."

"So, wait," he said, genuinely perplexed. "Is it vegan?"

It dawned on us both that if these companies are truly successful, then perhaps we will enter a post-vegan era in which the term ceases to be meaningful.

Chapter Five

The Vegan Mafia

If slaughterhouses had glass walls, everyone would be vegetarian.

—Paul McCartney

F rohman Anderson III had the good fortune of being born in Barrington, Rhode Island. The quaint town just a few miles southeast of Providence consistently ranks among the wealthiest in the state. The mansions that dot its seashores are occupied by descendants of those who made their wealth in manufacturing in the late nineteenth century. Today, that wealth is perpetuated by Ivy League educations and careers in finance, investing, and real estate.

Despite, or maybe because of, the privileges he enjoyed growing up, Anderson's parents went out of their way to imbue their son and his older sister with the values of duty, service, and honor. When Anderson got to Dartmouth College, just like his father and grandfather before him, he chose to concentrate in environmental studies. Like many millennials, Anderson was concerned about climate change, and he had been passionate about the topic since high school.

Dartmouth's program was mostly focused on regenerative agriculture, and especially how to use animals for land management. At the time, that kind of thinking seemed perfectly natural to Anderson, who grew up hunting and fishing at his family's cabin in New Hampshire. But he also happened upon another course called Food Ethics in the philosophy department. That was the first time he was faced with questions like: How does what we eat affect somebody else halfway around the world? Is it morally justifiable to eat animals? How does what we eat impact climate change? Questions that Anderson had never confronted before.

Around this time, Anderson became ill, and discovered that he had a severe case of Lyme disease, a condition common on the East Coast, especially in New Hampshire, where the ticks that carry it hitch rides on deer in dense forests. Sent home for months, he spent much of his recovery time engrossed in topics related to health and wellness. To his surprise, he discovered research on the benefits of a plant-based diet. He also learned about the environmental consequences of meat production. "I thought, this can't be real." The deeper he dug, the more convinced he became that factory farming is to blame for large-scale environmental collapse.

The new discoveries were difficult to absorb. "The way eating meat was always presented to me, it's like this natural thing. It was so integral to our history and culture, and even to our survival, so I thought it was justified." Then he met a couple his age who came from a similar background but had been avid vegans for years. He jokingly calls them his "vegan parents." "Dave and Cayla answered all my philosophical questions. When I began to think about it as an ethical issue then suddenly, bam, it hit me. I decided to stop eating animals."

There was only one problem: his family. Anderson had no idea how his parents, sisters, and fiancé (now wife) Grace, his high school sweetheart, would react. That Christmas, he decided to address the issue head on. As his mother Kimberly explained to me later, "Fro came to us and said, I don't want any presents. All I want for Christmas is for you to watch these documentaries (*Forks over Knives* and *Cowspiracy*) and give me the time to talk about them with you." To his complete astonishment, his parents called him the next day and announced, "Okay, how do we do this?" On Earth Day in

2016, the entire Anderson family pledged to become vegan and set out to explore how they could use their wealth to support the cause.

Not long after, Anderson happened to go to an impact investing event at Harvard University organized for children of wealthy families. "They were talking about how their family's wealth was being invested in renewable energy, water accessibility, and sanitation. The idea spoke to me. I realized you could invest and make value and wealth while doing good things in the world." Anderson had some experience investing. Back in college during a summer internship at Fidelity Investments, he entertained himself by reading about Tesla, his favorite company. Tesla was the first investment he ever made, even when many thought the company was on the edge of bankruptcy. "People totally wrote off electric vehicles. But I could see that the company was positioned to capture the fundamental inefficiencies of existing technologies and then scale them up."

Years later, Anderson realized that Tesla going up against the fossil fuel industry was analogous to the alternative protein companies going up against animal agriculture. As he delved more deeply in the space, one of the first things he noticed was that many of the early companies were funded by the same investors. With a little digging, Anderson found they were all part of a group called the Glass Wall Syndicate. He reached out to the organizer, a woman named Lisa Feria. To his surprise, she replied that the group was having an in-person meeting in two weeks at the Future Food Tech Conference in San Francisco, and he should come along. "I had no idea what I was doing, but I just thought, I need to book a plane ticket to San Francisco right now. I crashed on my friend's couch and went to the event and Lisa invited me to the dinner with everyone else. And that's where I met all these people who had been investing in this space for years and they all seemed to know each other. I felt very out of place, but I just soaked up the conversation and tried to figure out who was who."

When he got back to Providence, he thought about investing in a vegan cheese company he had heard of called NuMu. As a new vegan, he missed melt-in-your-mouth pizza slices and daydreamed about starting a vegan cheese company of his own. He emailed Feria to ask whether she had heard of NuMu, and Feria put out a notice to the Glass Wall members. "I got an email from a Chris Kerr, one of the guys I met in San Francisco." Anderson didn't know much about Kerr other than that he was the chief investment officer of a fund called New Crop Capital (now called Unovis Asset Management). "Chris said, 'You're too early. They're not ready yet.'" Instead, he invited Anderson to an event he was hosting in New York City.

Anderson took the train down from Providence and found himself in an apartment in Brooklyn at a tasting for what turned out to be a new vegan seafood company. "It was under the radar—a secret project Kerr was working on. Bruce [Friedrich] was there, and so was Mark [Langley], the managing partner. They wanted me to try the products, since all of them had been vegan for decades. They said, 'You've only been vegan for six months. We need you to tell us if this tastes like seafood.'" That same day, they asked Anderson whether he might want to invest in the company that would eventually become Good Catch (which makes plant-based "seafood"). Without quite realizing it at the time, Anderson had just met the Vegan Mafia.

I wish I could take credit for the term "Vegan Mafia," but I first heard about it in a CNBC article that borrowed the nickname from "PayPal Mafia," a group of Silicon Valley investors that included Peter Thiel (Founders Fund), Elon Musk (Tesla and SpaceX), and Reid Hoffman (LinkedIn), who got their start working on PayPal in the 1990s. Like many others who read the piece, I was fascinated to learn that the vegan movement was supported by a few wealthy investors. Although the movement as a whole receives scant funding compared to many other fields, it was still fascinating to learn about their motivations. But this was early in the days of the alternative protein landscape, and the investors didn't necessarily think of themselves as a cohesive network just yet.

The article mentioned names like Kyle Vogt, CEO of Cruise, a self-driving car technology company; Kevin Boylan, a former Wall Street trader who runs PowerPlant Ventures (now Groundforce Capital) along with T. K. Pillan, founder of Veggie Grill; Seth Bannon and Ela Madej, Y Combinator alumni and cofounders of the venture firm Fifty Years; Ryan Bethencourt, former cofounder of IndieBio, a biotech accelerator through which many of the alternative protein companies had their start; and Lisa Feria, CEO of Stray Dog Capital and the person who first introduced Anderson to the space.

One person not mentioned is Chris Kerr, who took Anderson under his wing. And yet, over time, it became clear that he was running much of the show. Kerr's background is hard to pin down, and over the years, I've come to suspect that this is intentional. When we first met back in 2017, he described himself as an entrepreneur. He was obviously a successful one, as he retired early. A lifelong animal lover, he was inspired to become vegan in 2002 by his wife, Kirsty, and today they live with about a dozen cats.

Kerr was disturbed by all forms of animal abuse, but the sheer scale of factory farming convinced him to focus his attention on food. Kerr's life mission is to "save a billion animals before I die." In 2007, Kerr began to work with the Farmed Animals division of the Humane Society of the United States (HSUS), but their fund failed to get off the ground before the market collapsed. It wasn't until a few years later that he got a call from Bruce Friedrich. "Bruce told me there was a private donor who had been giving money to sanctuaries and animal protection groups, but they weren't making much of a dent. They set up a trust to invest in companies, but they didn't have anybody to manage it."

Kerr had direct experience in the space, having scaled the Canadian cheese company Daiya early on. "I flew to Vancouver to see the vegan cheese product they were making in their oven and I told them, 'You need to get this on the market now.'" At the time, nobody believed there was a demand for plant-based cheese, but Kerr knew that there was pent-up demand not among vegans, but from lactose intolerants. He was convinced the market for dairy alternatives was untapped. He was right. In 2017, Daiya became an instant hit, and a few years later, it was acquired by the Japanese pharmaceutical giant Otsuka Pharmaceutical.

But when Friedrich came to him with the offer to run Unovis, Kerr declined, mostly because he didn't want to deal with the bureaucracy of running a nonprofit. Just then, one of his cats went missing. Searching for her day and night, Kerr thought, "Why am I putting so much energy into saving one animal, and yet not taking a job that could potentially save billions?" He called Friedrich and said, "I'm in." The initial fund held $25 million, to be deployed at $5 million a year—a puny amount for most funds, but substantial in the chronically underfunded animal protection movement. Their first check was for the plant-based meal delivery company Purple Carrot, and soon after, Beyond Meat, NuMu, New Wave, Kite Hill, Ocean Hugger Foods, and Miyoko's Creamery. "My sweet spot is growing a company from zero to maybe $5 million in sales. After that they outgrow me."

To their portfolio companies, Unovis was far more than a venture firm. Working in tandem with GFI, their intent was to shape the entire alternative protein industry into an attractive investment opportunity. Kerr was particularly fond of the Japanese concept of *keiretsu*, the practice of setting up a network of businesses with interconnected relationships and shareholdings to ensure collective success. "If you are going to be a food company, you need a good chef, a manufacturer, a distribution company, and a major retailer." But you also need social media. "We needed to get these products in front of the early adopters and let it cascade."

Good Catch, the company Anderson invested in early on, is a good example of the vegan *keiretsu* at work. Unovis recognized a "white space," a market opportunity to meet consumers' need for plant-based seafood. To create the product, they brought in brothers Derek and Chad Sarno, long-time vegan chefs who previously worked at Whole Foods Market, and a CEO from a branding agency, and then seed-funded the whole enterprise while persuading other investors to join the round.

I witnessed the efficacy of this system firsthand when I volunteered at the Good Catch booth as my ticket into ExpoWest, the biggest natural foods show in the industry in 2018. As I stood around offering plant-based tuna salad and crab cakes to passersby, I watched Kerr and the other investors make visits to the booths of their portfolio companies, meeting with current and potential investors and sampling new products. It seemed everyone knew each other—there were lots of fist bumps and smiles—and I had a distinct feeling that they weren't as much competitors as teammates on a much bigger mission.

Unovis took the same approach with cell-cultured meat. They were involved with Upside Foods early on, and when Upside debuted its famous meatball, they brought in Chef David Anderson of Madeleine Bistro in L.A., the former head chef at Eat Just. As Kerr told me, "This was a very expensive meatball, so I needed it to be done right." When it came time to attract media attention, "GFI helped us make sure the announcement came out in the *Wall Street Journal*, not *VegNews*," underscoring the importance of attracting mainstream appeal.

Like GFI, Unovis's "thesis" is the idea that vegan activists should be investing their time into making better meat. As Kerr says, "I was tired of hitting people over the head with the moral sword and trying to change hearts and minds. Obviously, we're abusing animals in some way or another every day, and the idea is, wouldn't it be great if we stopped doing that? I don't want to get caught in the delusion that we'll make the world vegan. But these companies will make change easier. The idea is to take animals out of the equation."

———

Lisa Feria is an unlikely vegan. Feria isn't, as she puts is, a "hippie in Birkenstocks from Berkeley." Born and raised in Puerto Rico, she moved to the mainland to study chemical engineering at Georgia Tech. Lisa's first job out of college was with General Mills, where she learned how products like Cheerios get made. She went on to get her MBA at the Booth School of Business at the University of Chicago, and afterward landed at Procter & Gamble as a business manager. Part of her job there was to monitor possible threats to portfolio companies, including campaigns by activist organizations like Greenpeace and PETA.

Feria spent hours watching footage of factory farming, looking for strategies to protect the brands' PR. But to her surprise, she found herself siding with the activists. "I remember watching a PETA video called *Meet Your Meat* and thinking, There's no way this is true. They must have found a company in some small town that's the worst of the worst." Diving in deeper, she realized how omnipresent animal abuse is across industries. "I'm participating in this cruelty," she realized. Feria found herself slowly giving up meat and eventually embracing veganism. "I think of myself as a very pragmatic, businesslike person, so to have such a visceral reaction of right and wrong was new."

The philosophy felt right in her heart, but Lisa knew it would pose professional problems. At first she tried to find a position in the company that would allow her to avoid clients whose businesses participated in animal cruelty, but it was nearly impossible, not only in food but in the cosmetics, pharmaceutical, and fashion industries as well. "At some point my professional life and my personal beliefs were on a collision course, so I was looking for something that would unite my business acumen and my personal principles and put those together in a way that was meaningful for the movement."

Around this time, a recruiter reached out to her, noticing her social media posts and guessing, correctly, that she was vegan. There was a job opening in Kansas at a venture capital fund called Stray Dog Capital. Vegan animal lovers Charles (Chuck) and Jennifer Laue had started Stray Dog to support companion animal charities, but they were looking to expand, with the help of a vegan CEO with expertise in business. "When I met Chuck and Jennifer, I thought, 'We're one hundred percent aligned with what we want to do in the world.'" Feria and her family decided to move to Kansas, and the Laues introduced her to people they knew through the board of directors at HSUS. Bruce Friedrich was one of them, and it was only years later that Feria realized that he was the person behind the PETA video that had entirely changed her life. "I remember telling him that at the GFI conference and he was surprised. I mean, he hopes his work will have that kind of impact."

The other person Feria was introduced to was Chris Kerr. Early on, Kerr helped her map out the key financial players in the nascent space. "We gathered this core group and started collaborating. We weren't competing, because we both wanted the whole space to succeed, so we put our personal egos aside and worked together." Before long, it became a challenge to keep everyone in the loop, and they felt the need to formalize the network. Feria volunteered to start a formal organization, and the Glass Wall Syndicate (GWS) was born, named after Paul McCartney's well-known line from a 2010 PETA video: "If slaughterhouses had glass walls, everybody would be vegetarian."

When I first met Feria back in 2017, a year after the Glass Wall Syndicate was born, it already had dozens of members and was growing quickly. A hodgepodge of heirs to family fortunes, foundations, and venture firms, these investors nevertheless shared a clear mission: getting animals out of the food system. Among the earliest members include Baleine & Bjorn Capital, set up by the heir of the Smarties Candy Company; Fifty Years, run by the husband-and-wife team from the "Vegan Mafia" CNBC article; and Blue Horizon Corporation, started by an enigmatic technology entrepreneur-turned-investor based in Switzerland.

As Feria explained, "The market is ripe for innovation, there was a lot of appetite for these companies, but people didn't have access to deal flow, and didn't know who to invest in. That's where we came in." Some of the investors were motivated by animal welfare or climate change, while others were in it purely for the money, seeing an opportunity to take a share of the behemoth animal agriculture industry. It didn't matter to Feria whether they were "mission-aligned" or not, because their investments helped legitimate the cause.

GWS sent monthly memos about investment opportunities, and twice a year everyone met either in New York or San Francisco to hear pitches from the most promising companies. Before long, big-name investors started noticing a pattern, the same firms popping up in deals across the alternative protein landscape. "There they were, Cargill, Danone, and General Mills," Kerr told me. "They all wanted to get into this space, and guess who knew more than anyone about it? Dinky little New Crop Capital [Unovis], because we were in all the deals, and they were wondering who the heck we were." When they started calling him and Feria, asking them for advice, they knew they were on a roll. "These companies are not going to sit down with PETA. We helped them to understand the space and why they should invest."

Over the last few years, the most significant investments in this space have been from high-profile investors like Bill Gates and Richard Branson, as well as multinational food conglomerates. Other new investors were drawn in for ideological reasons, such as Leonardo DiCaprio and *Titanic* director James Cameron and his wife, Suzy Amis Cameron. While in Los Angeles, I interviewed Amis Cameron at Lightstorm Entertainment Studios. The couple met on the set of *Titanic* and are both lifelong environmentalists. After watching the documentary *Forks over Knives*, she felt "betrayed that we had been lied to our whole lives about the best things to be eating for our health." That night she and her husband got rid of all of the animal products in their house. Eventually, Cameron and her sister Rebecca Amis opened the MUSE school, the first entirely plant-based school in the United States. James Cameron even turned his entire *Avatar* set vegan.

The pandemic year was tumultuous in every sense, but it was a boon for the alternative proteins sector. While meat companies faced historical shortages due to COVID-19 outbreaks among their vulnerable slaughterhouse workers, plant-based companies continued to grow. Of the $5.9 billion raised by alternative protein companies over the past decade, more than half was received during 2020 alone, with more than 160 deals made.[1] This figure represents all three pillars of the sector: plant-based ($2.1 billion),[2] cell-cultured ($360 million),[3] and fermentation ($590 million), signaling excitement around the "future of food."[4]

None of that would have happened if not for the Vegan Mafia. As Kerr put it, "We've got moles. We've got people of influence everywhere. Nothing happens in this space without us knowing about it ahead of time. Intelligence gathering is a large part of what we do in the investment world. It's a bit like the mafia in that we have people in high places that can subtly influence decisions." One time, I asked Kerr point-blank if he considers himself the Godfather of the Vegan Mafia. "You might call me the Dogfather, but the truth is, I'd rather not be widely known, because if I am, I'm far less effective."

———

The Vegan Mafia funds only a specific kind of product—what they call "direct replacements" for meat, dairy, and eggs. That means they are interested in products that replicate not only the flavor and texture of conventional products, but also their protein composition. The term "protein" comes from the Greek *proteios*, which means "of prime importance," and was first isolated in 1839 by a Dutch chemist, Gerardus Johannes Mulder. Mulder described protein as "unquestionably the most important of all known substances in the organic kingdom."[5] We have since learned that although protein is undoubtedly important, it's just one of a whole plethora of nutrients that are essential for health and well-being.

When someone finds out I follow a plant-based diet, almost inevitably they ask, *But where do you get your protein?* Sometimes the question is innocent enough, but other times it's uttered in an ominous tone, as though I'm about to disintegrate into thin air. I used to try to explain that protein deficiency is only a problem when there is caloric deficiency—which is why we barely ever see it in the West—but that seldom assuages the concern. In fact, research shows that the average adult in the United States gets far *more* protein than advised by dietary guidelines, but a fifth of adults still consider themselves to be protein deficient, and these worries drive consumer decisions about what to purchase for their families.[6]

The vegan movement has embraced this concern by framing their products as "alternative protein," an idea that resonates deeply with Silicon Valley's ethos of "techno-optimism." Some of these enterprises were founded at the same time as Airbnb and Uber, companies that saw the hotel and taxi industries as outdated and inefficient. Capitalizing on this idea, vegan entrepreneurs pointed to the technological "inefficiencies" of animal agriculture and aimed to "disrupt" the industry. This marketing tactic was so successful that even meat companies began getting into the game, knowing as they did that meat—especially processed red meat—suffered from negative press. Industry incumbents like Cargill and Unilever acquired plant-based companies, and Tyson Foods even trademarked the term "The Protein Company."

One narrative common among many founders and investors is that historically, technology has been a boon to animals. An example I heard often was how lamp oil replaced whale blubber as a source of light. In the nineteenth century—as memorably depicted in Herman Melville's *Moby-Dick*—whales were routinely hunted for their blubber, which was used for oil lamps and soap. As Josh Tetrick, founder of Eat Just, told me, "Why did people stop putting guys on a boat, giving them harpoons, and getting them to kill whales? It's not because there was a mass movement to save whales, but because we refined oil into kerosene." The hunting of whales declined considerably, possibly saving them from extinction. The other example I heard was the invention of the Henry Ford's Model T, the first mass-produced car, which displaced horses as the primary mode of transportation more effectively than the activists who pleaded for compassion.

Still, we need to stay vigilant about the win-win narratives of techno-logical promises. As Michael and Joyce Huesemann write in their book *Techno-Fix*, this rhetoric claims that "advanced technology will extricate us from an ever-increasing load of social, environmental, and economic ills."[7] Technology-based solutions tend to focus on fixing a narrow problem, without necessarily considering unintended consequences. Petroleum may have played a role in preventing the extinction of whales, but it's also respon-sible for oil spills that are toxifying the oceans today. Cars and airplanes may have liberated horses, but now their exhaust pipes contribute to global warming. As the food writer Warren Belasco writes in his book *Meals to Come: A History of the Future of Food*, "whatever their positions, the futur-ists who have received the greatest attention have been the ones with the loudest, most urgent and certain scenarios, even if they have turned out to be wrong."[8]

While altruistic motives are central to the ethos these companies espouse, we'd be remiss to overlook the financial incentives. Some founders admitted that having a moral stance makes for a good story to tell investors, and obviously, do-gooder narratives aren't specific to the alternative protein sector. But we must remember that these companies are still operating within the VC system, and that system has its flaws. The infamous case of Theranos, a blood testing company whose technology did not work despite claims by its CEO Elizabeth Holmes, is a testament to the perils of Silicon Valley. Whatever the fiasco may indicate about Holmes herself, her story is also a warning about the pressures of milestone timelines and investor demands.

While touring the headquarters of some of these companies, I often found myself thinking, *Shouldn't we just be eating whole plant foods, rather than going through an elaborate protein extraction process?* At least in part, it's because there's money to be made. As Marion Nestle observes astutely in *Food Politics*, "Many of the nutritional problems of Americans—not least of them obesity—can be traced to the food industry's imperative to encourage people to *eat more* in order to generate sales and increase income."[9] The idea of protein as "center-of-the-plate" reinforces the false belief that we all need more protein, and the race to "biomimic" animal-based foods means that healthful ingredients like chickpeas, beets, and carrots don't sound "food tech" enough to Silicon Valley investors.

Still, in a deeply imperfect food system, these solutions may be a necessary, if not sufficient, part of the desperately needed transition to something better in order to avert climate catastrophe.[10] In my mind, these products fit into a category I think of as "absurd solutions to absurd problems." Sure, it may be absurd to extract proteins from plants only to mimic the taste and flavor of proteins in animals. Then again, our current system is based on an even more absurd food chain. It begins with growing soy, corn, and wheat on hundreds of thousands of hectares of land. Then we feed those crops (many of which might otherwise be fed to humans) to animals, wasting their caloric potential. Finally, we try to scale that system to meet the impossibly rising demand for meat worldwide. Alternative proteins are often billed as unsustainable. But the real question should always be "Unsustainable compared to what?"[11]

No doubt, touring these companies left me inspired, but the experiences also left me with many questions that were only beginning to percolate at the back of my mind. They came to the surface when I arrived at Berkeley, the land of the "conscious omnivore."

Chapter Six

Let Them Eat Grass-fed Beef

Eat food, not too much, mostly plants.

—Michael Pollan

E dible Education is a famous class in the food world. It was started in 2011 at UC Berkeley by the celebrated food writer Michael Pollan and Alice Waters, founder of the iconic California "slow food" restaurant Chez Panisse. Eventually it was taken over by William Rosenzweig, cofounder of the Republic of Tea and founder of the Sustainable Food Initiative at Haas, Berkeley's business school. Every year, Rosenzweig and his co-leaders convene speakers from across the food movement, and the class is live-streamed free for anyone who wishes to join. Class topics are those you might expect to find at Berkeley, known for its emphasis on social justice and activism: organic farming, food safety, farm bill reform, farm-to-school initiatives, labor, food sovereignty, and a newly blossoming buzzword: regenerative agriculture.

I got to know Pollan while I was in graduate school at Harvard University, where he teaches part of the year. When I began looking for an institutional home where I could write this book, he suggested I reach out to Rosenzweig, who invited me to sit in on a live class of Edible Ed while I was in town. After a couple of days attending a conference in downtown San Francisco titled "The Future of Protein," it felt like quite a contrast to attend one called "The What, Why and How of Regenerative Agriculture." I had a vague sense that the term had something to do with sustainability and ecosystems, but at the time, I didn't know what, exactly.

I arrived at the amphitheater-style classroom and found a seat near the front. (This was a few weeks before the pandemic forced everyone online.) The class host began, "You may have heard industry leaders picking something that is the trend of the year. Pantone, for example, always picks a color of the year, and this year it's classic blue. Webster's Dictionary picked a word of the year last year, and it was 'they.' I feel like if the food and farming community picked a word, our word of the year would be 'regenerative.' I hear it all the time, and it's filled with so much excitement and buzz, but what does it really mean?" She went on to quote the definition from the class syllabus: "A system of farming practices and principles that does four things: increases biodiversity, enriches soil, improves watersheds, and enhances natural ecosystem services."[1]

The panel consisted of four guests: an ecologist and soil scientist, two vegetable farmers, and a rancher. Dr. Whendee Silver, an ecologist and biochemist, went first, opening her talk with a quotation from the recently released report by the Intergovernmental Panel on Climate Change (IPCC), which warned, predictably, about the dire condition of our planet. She emphasized that at this point, reductions in carbon emissions would not be sufficient to meet the goals set out by the Paris Agreement. She explained the bottom line: "The report is saying that emissions reduction is no longer sufficient to resolving the climate change problem. We have to remove CO_2 out of the atmosphere in addition to reducing emissions."

She went on to discuss the Marin Carbon Project, an effort to study carbon sequestration on ranches. One of the ranchers she works with was beside her on the panel: Loren Poncia of Stemple Creek Ranch. Poncia is a fourth-generation cattle rancher whose great-grandfather left Italy for the greener pastures of Marin County in 1897. The ranch is located off Tamales Bay, close by Point Reyes, a pristine piece of land that juts out into the Pacific

Ocean about an hour north of San Francisco that is known for its wild elk population. At the time Poncia and his wife inherited the farm, he had been working a day job in farmed animal pharmaceuticals. "Let's just say," he explained, "I learned a lot about what I didn't want to do."

When Poncia took over the family farm, he decided to reinvent the business, including getting their land certified organic. Slowly, they began rotating cattle, switching them to an exclusively grass-based diet, the natural foodstuff of cows. (Cows on factory farms are fed corn and soy feed.) Instead of trying to sell their beef to the highest bidder, they began to sell directly to consumers. They found a receptive market in affluent Marin County, where customers were willing to pay a premium for "grass-fed" and "grass-finished" products, a niche market that was only just emerging.[2]

The moderator asked Poncia about the negative press around beef: "Right now, there's this narrative that 'Beef is bad,' and *industrialized* beef is bad for the planet, but not *all* beef is bad. Can you tell us about your ranching practices and its climate impacts and why yours is better?"

"I love this topic," began Poncia, "I love to talk about fake meat and beef." The audience laughed and Poncia chuckled. "We have more customers daily who want to know what we're doing, and our sales have never been better. In the face of plant-based protein—or plant-based meat, as some people would have you call it—our sales are strong and growing, and I'm frankly not worried about those alternative meats because most are fast food. If you look at the ingredient list, go and have an Impossible Burger and there's ten things on the list. If you want to have a Stemple Creek burger, there's one ingredient, and it's regenerative beef. Plus, we're sequestering more carbon and we have data to prove it."

Excitedly, Poncia then showed before and after photos of his land on the overhead projector. "This is the front window of my parents' house looking out onto the creek when I was a child." The picture, apparently taken in 1990, shows a dry-looking landscape. Poncia flipped to an "after" photo of what the land looks like today. "This is it today," he said, proudly showing a lush green landscape. "It's full of life. I use these beasts"—up goes a picture of a happy-looking cow—"to try and mimic mother nature and what was going on in the Great Plains three or four hundred years ago with bison. They'd eat the grass in front of them, stomp on the ground below them, poop on the grass behind them, and it would regenerate the soil, building massive roots." More pictures comparing his lush green landscape to the yellow grasses of his neighbor just over the fence. "As people like us are becoming successful, our neighbors are starting to pile on."

When it came time for audience questions, one student asked a question that seemed to be present for many in the classroom: "Does your ranch sequester more carbon than your cows produce methane? I'm confused about whether it's a bigger impact for me not to eat meat or to focus more on where my food comes from."

"That's a great question," said Poncia, offering a surprisingly humble answer. "So far, from the initial data that we have on our ranch, we're net positive. We're sequestering about two pounds of carbon per pound of meat than we raise, but that's not the case with all of agriculture, and honestly, that data is a bit squishy right now. The land that our cattle are on right now is not tillable land, there's nothing else you can do with it. By grazing correctly—and even I sometimes don't do it perfectly—we're creating more biomass and pulling more carbon from the atmosphere, so we're building more soil. But the jury's still out. I would stay away from feedlot beef."

The mic was then passed to one of the farmers, a "seed keeper" named Kristyn Leach of Namu Farm. "I think sometimes we're told a plant-based diet is inherently better," she began. "But I'm going to slam Impossible Foods, since Loren already started it. The reality is that the problem of methane and greenhouse gases isn't only about the metabolism of a cow. It's about all these other industrial processes upstream that get us an overly processed plant-based food product. All the plastic that it's packaged in, and all the commodity crops processed in a factory. There's a lot of fuzzy math that's used in pitching these newfangled ideas, and I do think a plant-centered diet is great, and I should know because I grow vegetables, but simply eat beans from your local farmer. Eat delicious beef from Loren as opposed to eating the shiny new thing that's being dishonest in blaming an animal for methane production and not the processes that it's entrenched in."

The audience clapped approvingly, and there were laughs all around. "When I was young," chimed in Poncia, "people thought margarine was better for you. Ten years from now we'll be saying, *Remember when we thought Impossible was better for you than the real thing?* Don't get confused with the facts and just do what you think is right and know your farmer. It's that simple." My stomach sank. How was I supposed to write a book about veganism and alternative protein *here*?

———

Naively, I assumed that UC Berkeley, with its reputation as the birthplace of the Free Speech Movement of the 1960s and the farm-to-table movement of the '70s, would be a haven for veganism. Wasn't the Bay Area a leader in the alternative protein revolution? To my chagrin, I found that most of those passionate about food at UC Berkeley had little patience for what they often called the "vegan agenda," and much of their displeasure seemed linked to the buzzword "regenerative agriculture." As a freshly minted vegan, I found that their attitude filled me with a mix of dread and indignation, but also a genuine curiosity to understand what lay behind their skepticism.

I found out that the term "regenerative agriculture" was coined in the 1970s by Robert Rodale, an organic farmer, who declared, "The number one priority in regenerative organic agriculture is soil health."[3] Soil health is a defining priority of regenerative agriculture today, but the term also draws on principles from permaculture, also developed in the '70s by Bill Mollison and David Holmgren, as well as the concept of *holistic management* or *holistic grazing* developed by the controversial scientist and livestock farmer Allan Savory. (It's worth noting, of course, that regenerative practices have been used by indigenous land stewards for millennia.)

As far as I could see, the food community couldn't quite settle on a satisfactory definition, and I noticed disagreements and discrepancies in how it was used by academics, farmers, activists, and certainly the leaders of companies both big and small.

Another person who noticed these inconsistencies was Peter Newton, a professor at the University of Colorado, Boulder. Newton teaches an introductory course on environmental studies, and a couple of years ago, many of his students began to ask him to define the term in a succinct way. Newton didn't have a clear answer, so he did what academics do when they don't know—he did a study. In an extensive literature review, Newton and his colleagues tracked the term and how it was used in over two hundred academic journals. About half failed to define it, while the other half referred to a kaleidoscope of principles and practices.

Newton and his colleagues placed the existing definitions into three buckets: process-based, outcome-based, and both. The process-based definitions focus solely on what regenerative farmers do—plant cover crops, reduce tillage, integrate livestock, and so on. The outcome-based definitions focus on measurable achievements like the amount of carbon sequestered or improvements in water quality, but the *way* farmers got there mattered less than the result. The third bucket combined elements of both, suggesting that both the *how* and the *why* matter.

For some, including Rodale, regenerative agriculture means improving soil health, while for others, it means engaging in practices that prevent soil erosion such as no-tilling (leaving topsoil in place) and cover cropping (planting crops in between seasons). For still others, regenerative agriculture inherently means incorporating grazing ruminants (most often cows but sometimes goats) into the farming practice. The term is also used in a generalist way to refer to any kind of farming that promotes human health, food access, or food safety. Some highlight small-scale systems and community development, regardless of farm size. A minority even use the term "regenerative" synonymously with "profitable," but most see that as a problematic cooptation. Others flat out reject the term, preferring others like "agroecology," "real organic," and "regenerative organic." Some point out that practices in harmony with the land have been employed by indigenous farmers all over the world since the beginning of agriculture, and that it's only in the last few decades that the idea has been turned into a buzzword.

Not surprisingly, the debate between those advocating for regenerative agriculture and those advocating for veganism centers on the role of animals in agriculture. Many vegans believe that all animals must be taken out of agriculture entirely, while regenerative agriculturalists see them as indispensable to a healthy ecosystem. This rhetoric is often framed as "It's not the cow, it's the how" by advocates from the Savory Institute, started by Allan Savory. A Zimbabwe-born agriculturalist, Savory advocates for "holistic grazing," where the idea is to rotate cattle in a way that mimics the grazing patters of large herbivores (like bison) that used to roam the world's grasslands. In a 2013 TED talk, Allan Savory claimed that this type of grazing "can take enough carbon out of the atmosphere and safely store it in the grassland soils for thousands of years." The 2020 Netflix film *Kiss the Ground* claimed that by increasing soil organic matter on agricultural soils, regenerative livestock systems could sequester enough carbon to negate all current emissions.

Such claims have been widely disputed.[4] In 2017, scholars at Oxford University conducted a meta-analysis and found that grass-fed livestock offers a way to sequester carbon only under very small, time-limited, and reversible conditions, which are outweighed by the greenhouse gases that farms emit. Dr. Tara Garnett of Food Climate Research Network (FCRN), lead author of the Oxford study, concluded: "Grass-fed livestock are not a climate solution. Grazing livestock are net contributors to the climate problem, as are all livestock. Rising animal production and consumption, whatever the farming system and animal type, [are] causing damaging greenhouse gas release and contributing to changes in land use. Ultimately, if high-consuming individuals and countries want to do something positive for the climate, maintaining their current consumption levels but simply switching to grass-fed beef is not a solution. Eating less meat, of all types, is."[5]

Despite this research, the basic idea that it's not meat that's the problem, but how it's raised, has gained as much traction as veganism in recent years, if not more. One of the outspoken defenders of beef is the former environmental lawyer turned cattle rancher Nicolette Hanh Niman, who also lives in the Bay Area. In her aptly titled book *Defending Beef*, Niman tells the story of how she began to change her mind about meat when she married her husband, Bill Niman of Niman Farms. Unlike many vegetarians, as an environmental lawyer, Niman had direct exposure to factory farms and worked on campaigns against the pollution caused by industrial meat consumption.

But when she moved to her husband's ranch in Bolinas, California, she learned more about the realities of farming. She began to believe that if cows are allowed to roam and eat diverse natural grasses and shrubs like their wild ancestors, they will enhance natural diversity, restore soils, and capture carbon in the process. Since their farm uses no chemicals or antibiotics, the meat is more healthful for people too. The cows would also be happier, since they are able to express their natural behavior, as they cannot on feedlots.

Reading Niman's book, I found myself agreeing with many of her points, especially her critiques of the business-as-usual way of raising beef on factory farms. I also agreed with her concerns about ultraprocessed foods as being the culprit behind poor health. Still, for me the book raised many more questions than it answered. Setting aside my animal welfare concerns, I had my doubts about whether the "grass-fed beef" solution was truly scalable, or environmentally sustainable. Not only were some of the claims quite bold, but they seemed to downplay the complexities. They also seemed impractical—the regenerative beef I've seen at farmers markets in the Bay Area is very expensive compared to the typical feedlot beef at Safeway or Kroger. I knew I needed to talk to an expert. Luckily, I knew just the right one, who happened to be an old friend from graduate school.

———

Matthew Hayek and I met not, as many who know us both assume, working on various plant-forward initiatives at Harvard, but at the checkout line at Market Basket, a grocery store in Somerville, Massachusetts, that boasts cheap good-quality produce (naturally, it's a favorite haunt of students on a budget). It was around my birthday, and I decided that I wanted to host a dinner party in my tiny apartment, serving everyone an appetizer of pumpkin soup in individually carved miniature pumpkins. It was just the kind of ambitious idea I had in the early days of my enthusiasm for the plant-based way of life. Hayek noticed the dozen pumpkins in my cart and couldn't resist asking me what I planned to make. When I said pumpkin soup, he offered recipe ideas, and our friendship was born.

While I chipped away at my dissertation on the rise of the vegan movement, traveling to conferences or doing fieldwork at company headquarters, Hayek spent his days as an environmental engineer either in the lab or in the actual field, climbing old growth trees in the Amazon rainforest to collect samples of greenhouse gas emissions. Once, on a trip to France to attend a conference, we spent a week trying out all the vegan restaurants in Paris, and then a weekend cooking up a plant-based feast for friends in Normandy with produce from a lush garden.

After grad school, Hayek accepted a postdoctoral position as an Animal Law and Policy fellow at Harvard Law School, where he focused on greenhouse gas emissions from agricultural activities. A couple of years later he landed a position as a professor of environmental studies at New York University, where he began zeroing in on the environmental impact of food consumption. Few scholars were doing this kind of work at the time, and his rigorous and path-breaking research began to gain attention.

One of the papers that got Hayek's work on the map was on grass-fed beef; specifically, on the implications of a nationwide shift to that model of agriculture. The title of the paper says it all—"Nationwide Shift to Grass-Fed Beef Requires Larger Cattle Population,"[6] co-authored with Rachel D. Garrett at Boston University. At the time they started the paper, the term "grass-fed beef" was just beginning to become a buzzword, and Hayek wondered what this kind of agriculture would mean at scale. He was skeptical that grass-fed would be a sustainable solution, since he remembered the findings of a famous United Nations report titled "Livestock's Long Shadow," which showed that when cattle graze on pastures, they have a much bigger impact on greenhouse gas than when they are concentrated on factory farms.

Hayek and his colleague set out with a simple question: If the entire country transitioned to grass-fed beef, how many cattle would need to be raised to meet current demands? Based on data from the U.S. Department of Agriculture, they calculated that we'd need to raise 30 percent more cattle than we do now if we moved toward an entirely grass-fed system for all beef. That's because cattle eating their natural diet of grass take longer to fatten up and don't gain nearly as much weight as those on feedlots, who are fed a diet of corn and soy. Such a drastic increase would have monumental consequences for greenhouse gas output.

We already use a third of available land to raise cattle for food. If we were to use all of that land for grass-fed beef, then we'd be able to produce only about two-thirds of the current meat we consume. That switch would also result in a 41 percent increase in methane emissions—more cows, more emissions. These metrics are conservative, since they don't even consider the projections that meat consumption will *rise*, not fall, in the next few decades.

Even if we were to agree that eating more grass-fed beef is a good thing, I wondered, wouldn't we be sacrificing land that could be used for other purposes? I knew that livestock already occupy four-fifths of global farm-land[7] and contribute somewhere between 14 and 30 percent of green-house gas (GHG) emissions.[8] How would *more* grazing livestock solve that problem? It turned out that Hayek had written another paper that addressed that exact question, called "The Carbon Opportunity Cost of Animal-Sourced Food Production on Land."[9] In the paper, published in the presti-gious journal *Nature Sustainability*, Hayek and his colleagues ask what would happen to the carbon if we were to use agricultural land differently (putting aside economic questions such as the impact on livelihoods of those in the current agricultural sector). They calculated the carbon emissions from all food production and found that the carbon costs of producing beef and sheep are ten times higher than plant-based alterna-tives like tofu or tempeh.

The most surprising result is that if everyone were to shift to a plant-based diet worldwide, that would translate to a reduction in agricultural land use of 75 percent, allowing for rewilding and restoration of habitats. Rewilding has been shown to create meaningful carbon sinks and restore biodiversity, as wild animals nourish soil, draw carbon from the atmosphere, prevent wildfires, and in general create more resilience in our ecosystems.[10]

In fact, according to a well-cited study published in *Science*, a wholesale shift to a vegan diet worldwide would be the only way we could potentially stay below 1.5 degrees of warming, the tipping point beyond which we are headed for climate catastrophe.[11] The article shows that even if we don't all "go vegan," if we at least follow an "EAT-Lancet diet"—essentially a Mediterranean-style diet with less meat—there would still be a substantial impact. In the end, getting off meat and dairy will not solve our climate issues—we still need to get off fossil fuels—but doing so would drastically reduce the climate impacts of our food consumption.

Given that the reduction is unlikely to happen purely as a result of people's dietary choices, for Hayek, alternative proteins are perhaps the only truly viable solution at scale. As he told me in one of our conversations, "I think we can get people to consider lentils and farro bowls and whole plant foods, but I think we also need food that looks like an entrée to most people. We need cutting-edge meat substitutes that can be an effective gateway drug to getting off the amount of meat we eat." Hayek pointed out that as much as soy is a maligned food, making convincing soy-based alternatives to chicken and pork, for example, would ultimately lead to less acreage of soy planted, since most of that soy is currently going toward animal feed. "We need research into a diverse array of legume crops. The solution is research into these other proteins, not large-scale grass-fed beef. It's an agricultural harm reduction approach."

Hayek's idea of a "harm reduction agriculture" makes sense to me. The truth is that I found both the "future of food" fantasy of Silicon Valley and the utopian vision of grass-fed-beef-for-all at UC Berkeley to be unrealistic. One is based on the idea that you can replace all meat consumption with new technologies. The other assumes that everyone can support their local farmers, regardless of where they may live (or perhaps that everyone lives in a place like the Bay Area). I began to envision a middle path between the two—one in which we focus on new and alternative technologies but also consider how to move toward a system of agriculture that is based on diversity, polycropping, and systemic transformation.

The reality is that while plant-based products (and even cell-cultured meat, which often includes plant-based components) have the potential to displace animal agriculture, they don't often offer solutions to problems in agriculture writ large. One way they could be improved is if they contributed to diversification. As is, humans cultivate less than 1 percent of the estimated edible plant species that exist in the world.[12] For millennia, we have focused on improving the productivity of a smaller number of existing crops rather than increasing crop diversity. That has created a food system that is susceptible to potentially catastrophic losses due to disease and climate change.

It is precisely this industrialized food system that the advocates of regenerative agriculture are trying to resist. To the regenerative agriculturalists, the vegan techno-meat is yet another instance of the business-as-usual commodity monoculture agricultural system, simply sans animals. That, in essence, is what the Edible Ed participants were booing that day in the classroom. It's a solution that goes against all that regenerative agriculture stands for, which is diversity, resilience, and soil health for generations to come.

But what if we could harness the regenerative agriculture revolution to enhance the plant-based movement? What if we could integrate more regenerative agriculture practices—like cover crop rotation, tillage, and soil amendments—that don't use animals at all? These practices exist, and as an article in *Frontiers in Climate*[13] has shown, they are far more effective in improving soil's ability to capture carbon.

It's strange, if you think about it, that vegans and regenerative agriculturalists would have so much beef with each other, since their visions are not only compatible but in fact offer many of the most exciting opportunities to build a better food system. Vegans want a vast reduction (if not elimination) of meat consumption; regenerative agriculturalists want a system in which animals live better lives, and that vision is only feasible in a world where we vastly reduce our meat consumption. Far less (think once a week), but better, meat, and better livelihoods for farmers too, but only if consumers are willing to pay more. Let's not forget that both sides of the debate have a common enemy—factory farming—and it is in this field, it seems to me, that we should meet.

Ultimately, it's up to us to regulate, control, and utilize technologies in the best ways we can, with the right political incentive structure. We need policies that target meat consumption specifically through taxation, nudges to plant-based diets, and support for regenerative alternatives. If some meat consumption is reduced through plant-based or cell-cultured meat grown with renewable energy, that extra land could be used for planting more diverse crops for human consumption, for experimenting with climate-resistant crops that could be of use in the future, or even for rewilding efforts to increase biodiversity. These are all choices that we can make as a society.

After my conversation with Hayek, I thought back to the Edible Ed class on regenerative agriculture, and I began to wonder what the class's founder would think of this debate. Many of these same questions guided Michael Pollan on the journey that would become *The Omnivore's Dilemma*, a book that established him as one of the most authoritative voices on food. I was curious to hear his thoughts on the new "future of food" offered by vegans, and whether it could be reconciled with the vision of regenerative agriculture burgeoning in the Bay area and beyond.

———

I first met the iconic writer at a fireside chat at Harvard University's Radcliffe Institute for Advanced Study, where he was a visiting scholar for a year. Pollan was set to converse with Richard Wrangham, the anthropologist best known for arguing that cooking with fire led to our evolution. Pollan had just written about Wrangham's work in his latest book, *Cooked*. After the discussion, I came up to Pollan and asked him about his views on veganism. Even though this was several years ago, I remember Pollan's response as though it was yesterday: "I think it's great to eat plants, but tell me, why are vegans so self-righteous?"

Over a few years, our paths crossed only occasionally, and sometimes spontaneously (once at the North Berkeley organic farmers market), but slowly we bonded over a shared interest in food, nature, and consciousness, and I eventually became one of his research assistants. The first time I came over to his house in Berkeley, we sat at his dining table with cups of green tea, admiring his front garden. Before we even began talking, his wife, Judith, an artist, came downstairs and announced, "Did you know we've basically been vegan for months now?" I looked over at her husband and he acknowledged her comment. "It's true. We still eat fish from time to time, but I don't talk about it much." Clearly, Pollan's thinking had evolved since we met, and I wanted to know how. Luckily for me, Pollan agreed to an interview.

In truth, Pollan has always been an advocate of a plant-forward diet. As he famously advised, "Eat food. Not too much. Mostly plants." This mantra, which opened his *New York Times* article "Unhappy Meals"[14] in 2007, took on a life of its own. "I joke that it's going to be inscribed on my tomb," he quipped. "It turned out the word *mostly* was the most controversial. The meat people were like, what do you mean by *mostly*? The vegans were like, why not *exclusively*? It's a squishy word and people find it offensive on both sides. For me, it was a summary of the science that I read that clearly stated you are better off eating mostly plants, but there's no reason not to have any meat at all. That squishy word ended up being very useful."

But I wondered what "mostly" meant for Pollan personally these days. "You can't get too close to the meat industry without losing your taste for at least industrially produced meat. I was moving in the direction of plants already, except for special occasions like cooking a whole hog in the fire pit," he said, pointing out to his front yard. I recalled the scene from the *Cooked* documentary, in which Pollan roasts a hog he hunted in the Marin headlands. But more recently, Pollan and his wife follow a more "veganish" diet. Pollan doesn't like the word "vegan" because of its absolutism. "Every now and again you might slip, or you might choose to participate in a meal [that includes meat]. But that doesn't mean you have to get off the band-wagon entirely." Just as when we first met, Pollan doesn't like the self-righteousness, but he sees the value of veganism for both health and his mounting concerns about climate change.

Pollan isn't alone in wanting to embrace the benefits of eating plants without subscribing to the ideology. Many people prefer "plant-based" or "plant-centered" to "vegan." Some actively want to distance themselves from the "vegan" label and its associated stigma and stereotypes. Others want to distinguish a more health-oriented vegan diet. Still others use the terms interchangeably, or at times together. I fall in that category. For me, the term "vegan" refers to my philosophical stance, while "plant-based" emphasizes my concern with health and the ethics of how food is grown. If I had to describe myself, I'd say a I'm a whole food plant-based vegan who cares how her food is grown. But clearly, that's a mouthful.

This fuzziness creates flexibility, but also confusion. Sometimes "plant-based" refers to a diet that simply excludes animal products. Other times, it signifies a diet that excludes animal products and is concerned with health, usually free of sugar, salt, and sometimes even oil. And of course, the term is also used by the alternative protein industry to refer to "edible foodlike substances" (as Pollan would say) that replicate animal-based products but ultimately belong in the processed food category. With the rise of the term "plant-based," some ethically motivated vegans judge others for not doing it for the "right" reasons—which is exactly the moral purity that turns Pollan off. Many of these vegans see the health motivation as "selfish" and suspect "plant-based" eaters of being uninterested in the fate of animals and therefore less likely to remain committed.

For Pollan, like for many others, the "veganish" transition hasn't been easy. Besides having to relearn how to cook, the most challenging part is eating out, especially at other people's homes. By now, he's figured out how to order vegan pizzas at the Cheese Board Collective, one of his favorite Berkeley haunts, and even asks for a vegan meal when he goes to Chez Panisse. But he still hasn't gotten over the awkwardness of offending friends. "We're now in an era when nobody ever goes to a dinner party without being asked about their dietary restrictions, so it's better than it used to be, but still, I remember when someone was coming over and announced they were vegan I was having a panic attack in the kitchen. Like, what are we going to make? No, can't make that, it has some butter in it. I understand how people feel. It's got a social cost."

The transition has also been tricky given Pollan's reputation for supporting the grass-fed movement. "I still support the kind of small-scale animal agriculture I wrote about. I continue to believe that they're offering the right alternative to industrialized meat. But I have had one or two ranchers who were clearly annoyed with me." He told me about a butcher shop down the street where he used to get grass-fed beef. "I was recently in touch with the owner and his wife asked me, 'Why haven't we seen you lately?' When I said I've been eating a plant-based diet, she got upset. I don't want to disappoint people I still support."

Pollan told me that this butcher shop, which caters to the conscious omnivores of North Berkeley, had been a target for vegans from the Direct Action Everywhere (DxE) movement, who protested outside the establishment for months. Hoping to reach a truce, the owner reluctantly agreed to hang a MEAT IS MURDER sign outside his window. To Pollan, the activists' efforts were misguided, especially given how carefully the owner was sourcing his meat from local ranches. "What did they accomplish? Cognitive dissonance in the minds of a few conscious Berkeley meat consumers?"

Pollan has a point. While publicity stunts can be an important tactic for activists to highlight the ethical concerns around animal agriculture even on "humane" farms, they sometimes miss the broader point—and the opportunity—to bring more people into the fold. To me at least, it seems clear that perfection should not be a criterion for participation in the vegan movement, and that a harm reduction approach like the one Hayek described will take us a lot further. "We're so all or nothing, especially when it comes to food," Pollan observed. "I think the best we can hope for is reduction in meat consumption." And that, it turns out, is what the vegans and regenerative agriculturalists have in common.

———

As I was finishing this book, I had the privilege of spending a few days at the Mesa Refuge, a writing retreat overlooking Tamales Bay in Point Reyes, where Pollan wrote part of *The Omnivore's Dilemma*. On my first day there, I happened to pick a hiking trail near the Drakes Estuary, a place of astonishing, serene beauty. Hiking down through the eucalyptus grove and passing over the grasslands overlooking the estuary, I suddenly came upon a cow—a huge black creature blocking the trail. Silhouetted against the backdrop of the stunning landscape, it embodied the life most people imagine of the meat they eat, and yet this cow is the bovine equivalent of the one percent.

A couple of hundred years ago, these lands were occupied by Indigenous Coast Miwok people who had been living there for generations. But then ranchers took over these "marginal lands" in a pattern that the historian Joshua Specht has shown to have played out all over the country with devastating consequences.[15] Ever since, ranchers in this region—including Loren Poncia's ancestors, whose farm is nearby—have obtained special protections.

As the scholars Jan Dutkiewicz and Gabriel Rosenberg explain in a piece called "The Myth of Regenerative Ranching,"[16] when the National Park Service, which manages Point Reyes National Park, acquired these "historic" ranches, they allowed them to continue commercial operations for twenty-five years. That time horizon continues to be extended, despite the fact that the cattle pose a significant risk to native wildlife, including the local tule elk.

Ranchers have engaged in various practices that threaten the elk population, including culling (killing) members of the herd and putting up fences that block the elk from reaching fields for grass and drinking water, which has led to widespread deaths during droughts.[17] For at least as long as the Miwok people inhabited the lands, elk have grazed the seashore, living in ecological harmony with their human neighbors, yet now ranchers claim that the presence of their cattle on these lands is "natural" and the NPS still protects the cattle, not out of concern for animal welfare but due to their status as commodities, and refuses to protect these lands as Miwok heritage sites. Furthermore, the ranches leach *E. coli* bacteria runoff from manure into surrounding soil and streams. In 2022, a new lawsuit was issued by several environmentalist organizations to contest the National Park Service's privileging of the ranching industry over public and indigenous interests.

Seeing the cattle grazing, I pondered the deeper question. What, exactly, does "natural" mean? Products on shelves are said to contain "natural flavorings," which sound harmless enough, yet they are chemically produced. We used to make cheese with rennet harvested from the stomach lining of cows, but now we use precision fermentation to create the enzyme biochemically in a lab. For millennia we hunted animals for food, then for centuries we raised them on agricultural lands, and now we are engineering meat in bioreactors. The cows might look happy, but their fenced-in predator-free life is hardly natural, and has had an outsize negative impact on this landscape.

Advocates of regenerative agriculture often paint a romantic pastoral image of animal husbandry that doesn't quite square with reality. I hardly ever hear them grappling with the deep moral implications of eating animals, no matter how good a life they live, or acknowledging that cattle have been present on these lands for only a few generations. They may believe that raising cattle on their pastures is good for the soil, but they bring those animals' lives to an end believing it's natural and morally justifiable to do so. The subtle assumption of dominion still lurks in their rhetoric—*Animals are here for us to use.*

The bottom line is this: Regenerative agriculture presents a compelling solution to the problem of factory farming. However, it's not a silver bullet, just as veganism is not the silver bullet it often claims to be. We need to figure out how to vastly reduce meat consumption, not perpetuate a storybook narrative about rolling green pastures and happy cows. But rather than focusing on the simplistic dichotomy implied by the student in the Edible Ed classroom that day—*Is it better to stop eating meat or eat only grass-fed beef?*—I instead wanted to know, what would a truly regenerative, plant-based food system look and taste like, and what are the barriers to making it a reality?

Chapter Seven

From the Ground Up

Eating with the fullest pleasure—pleasure, that is, that does not depend on ignorance—is perhaps the profoundest enactment of our connection with the world.

—Wendell Berry

When Emma Jagoz was a child, her father wrote a book for his four children called *Moon Valley Stories*. In the stories, each child had a superpower. Jagoz's gift was the ability to communicate with plants and animals. She had a great big red barn and a greenhouse where all the plants and animals lived together in harmony. She even had a pig named Minerva, for whom she once threw a birthday party. Her father's musing about Jagoz's gift turned out to be a prophecy. Three decades later, Jagoz does indeed have a big red barn and several greenhouses. A vegan farmer, she is building a world that would make the story version of herself proud. "My secret mission," she told me the first time we spoke, "is to prove that farming doesn't have to rely on animal inputs."

Jagoz's parents became vegetarians in the 1970s. Her father was influenced by his brother, who became an ethical vegan, and her mother by a stint in the Peace Corps. When they had children, they began raising them on a vegetarian diet. They eventually began eating meat again when their son refused to eat vegetables, but they gave each child a choice about what kind of diet to eat. Although she was only three at the time, Jagoz chose to remain a vegetarian. She has never tasted meat in her life. "My mom always tells this story about how once when she asked me what I wanted for my birthday dinner, I said peas and carrots."

Yet it was not until her early twenties, when she became pregnant with her first child, that Jagoz decided to embrace veganism. "Like a lot of expecting mothers, I got obsessed with my diet." She learned that folic acid is essential to healthy brain development and began spending most of her grocery budget on organic arugula. Soon enough she decided to grow her own on her apartment balcony. "I got the gardening bug. It was deeply satisfying to me be able to grow not only for myself, but for my baby's health." Soon, Jagoz wanted to grow more, a lot more. She asked her parents if she could use the land outside their house in suburban Balti-more and moved back home to tend to it. Eventually, she learned to can tomatoes, pickles, and beets, and had such a surplus of vegetables that she began giving some away to friends and neighbors. "It dawned on me that maybe I could start a business."

Even if it may have seemed that she was fulfilling her destiny, the journey to becoming a farmer wasn't an easy one. When Jagoz moved back home permanently, she was pregnant with her second child, a daughter. Farming while pregnant was incredibly challenging, and at the time she didn't have any help. Her former husband (they've since divorced) was commuting to D.C. for work. She didn't have enough land, nor labor, but she is an incred-ibly hard worker, and she's scrappy. "I made compost from free things I found—you know, a neighbor's grass clippings, raked-up leaves, or the horse manure I took off people's hands in the neighborhood."

With two young children in tow, hauling her food to the weekend farmers market was out of the question. Instead, she started with a community-supported agriculture (CSA) model. In her first year, 2012, she fed twelve families from a quarter acre on her parents' property. She quickly realized that she wanted to grow certain crops that needed more space—melons, potatoes, and winter squash—and to do that she'd need more land. She began bartering with neighbors for pieces of land in exchange for a CSA share. By the end of 2019, she had fifteen acres across six properties, two bordering her parents' property and three within a half hour's drive. Transporting labor and equipment (not to mention children) across all the lots was a logistical nightmare that left her completely exhausted by the day's end. But all the while, she was driven by a sense of social justice around access to good-quality, nutritious food. "If you don't have your health, you don't have anything, and right now, people's health is being denied to them through government subsidies for non-food food." A self-described "action person," she felt empowered by growing food not only for herself and her family, but for others in her community.

Jagoz and I met through our mutual mentor Will Rosenzweig at UC Berkeley. Rosenzweig had invited her to give a talk at Plant Futures, a class I helped to start with my friend Samantha Derrick. I found Jagoz's talk about her journey completely captivating. Even though I had a spent a decade studying food, it was from an academic perch. I had never "gotten my hands dirty," so to speak. In other words, I knew next to nothing about how to actually grow and produce food. I had many questions for Jagoz, no doubt many of them naïve, but she generously agreed to let me come visit and see the farm for myself.

———

I came to see Moon Valley Farm—forty acres of farmland near Chesapeake Bay, named after her father's stories—one Friday in late October. It was an unseasonably warm autumn day, but the air had a crispness that foreshadowed the cold weather to come. As Douglas and I made our way through D.C., we passed desolate reminders of the way most people in this country habitually eat. A McDonald's here, a 7-Eleven over there, a Charlie's Cheesesteaks in between. The sight was depressing, and Jagoz's words about "non-food food" ran through my mind.

As we made our way to the outskirts, the landscape of fast food joints was gradually replaced by rural flatness occasionally dotted with houses and farms. The fall foliage was a symphony of reds, oranges, yellows, and greens. By the time we turned onto Jagoz's long driveway about an hour later, we were surrounded by green and yellow pastures. At the top of the slightly upwardly slanted property stood a red brick house with white columns. Jagoz lives here with her children, two dogs, a cat, and her parents, who moved in with her in retirement. Her dad had recently suffered a brain injury, and between his condition, her divorce, the loss of a business partner, and the pandemic, it had been an intense few years.

Immediately to the left of the house stands a great big red barn, just like the one in *Moon Valley Stories*. Out front on the expansive field are five high white tunnels—two for seedlings and three for produce. The tunnels shield her growing environment from the elements, dust, and pests, allowing her to extend her season. With climate change making the weather (especially rain) far more unpredictable each year, Jagoz knew they would be a solid investment in her business.

We parked our rental car and went looking for Jagoz, who turned out to be in one of the tunnels. It was only nine in the morning, but she had already been up for four hours. She was dressed in an EAT MORE KALE T-shirt, flannel shirt, hiking pants, and big work boots, looking the part. Generously, she took the rest of the morning and early afternoon off to show us around, accompanied by Minnie, a tiny black-and-white-spotted dog who trotted along behind her.

We started the tour in the storage unit, which the scrappy Jagoz had built herself. It contained two large walk-in coolers, one very cold and the other just chilly, for different kinds of produce. Some produce, like beets, can last for weeks, while others, like greens, must be sold quickly, but the coolers buy her time. A big whiteboard hung in between, listing all the restaurants they sold to that week. I mentally took a note to ask Jagoz for a recommendation of where we should try her food in the city. More than a hundred of the best local farm-to-table restaurants between D.C. and Baltimore source from her farm, among others.

Jagoz's original dream was to offer CSA members all the components of a well-rounded plant-based diet all on her own, but the upfront costs were far too high to invest in the technology she needed to make that a reality. Growing beans, for example, is an entirely different process from growing vegetables. When beans are harvested, they need to be cleaned thoroughly and shelled. Jagoz can grow beans without a problem, but cleaning "bean schmutz" and shelling at scale is impossible for her right now, whereas it's much easier for a farmer nearby. In her entrepreneurial way, Jagoz instead recruited other farmers in her community to become part of her CSA offer. Today, the farm boxes she sells include her vegetables along with mushrooms, beans, grains, and sourdough bread—as well as eggs and honey (though she doesn't eat them herself)—that her team home-delivers to her customers.

From the coolers we returned to the high tunnels to check out the ginger and turmeric, two of the most popular crops Jagoz is currently harvesting. The rows were waist high, filled with fresh bulbs: the ginger yellowish and pink, the turmeric light orange and fleshy. Jagoz explained that this is what ginger and turmeric look like before they reach maturity and dry out. I had tasted fresh ginger and turmeric only once before, back when I lived in Boston and biked down to buy provisions from the only organic stand at the Copley Square Farmers Market. They are a rare find, so chefs are excited about Jagoz's harvest.

We left the high tunnels for the fields out front, where Jagoz grows her brassicas, including kale, turnips, and kohlrabi, which are from the same plant family. Jagoz encouraged us to try some. I reached for the delicate white turnips, their little green heads of hair peeking out of the soil. I brushed off some of the dirt and bit in. Deliciously crunchy, they had a mild sweetness and creaminess I didn't expect from a vegetable. "Have you ever tasted fresh kohlrabi?" Jagoz asked. She bent down and pulled out a bulb I had seen at the farmers market but never ventured to try. She took out a pocketknife and skinned it, cutting the inside into pieces. It looked, and tasted, like a broccoli stem. "A lot of our CSA members have no idea what to do with kohlrabi, but I love it." Jagoz often has to educate her customers on how to use her produce, since they don't always get to choose what comes in the box. "I wish someone would just teach people how to eat vegetables."

We continued down the field, Minnie prancing behind us. At one point, as we tasted fresh peppers arranged in rows by heat level, Minnie suddenly decided to show off her hunting chops. But she quickly lost the trail of a field mouse scurrying below our feet and skittered off in the wrong direction. Jagoz pulled on her collar to point her the right way, but Minnie couldn't see the mouse that was obvious to us all. "To be fair, this is new for her. She's transitioning from being a pet to being a field dog with a job on the farm."

We continued our ramble through Jagoz's farm, stopping here and there to smell, taste, and ask questions. Jagoz led us up the hill, behind the house and barn, toward the herb garden. "One of the things I've learned as a farmer is that aromatherapy is real," she commented. As we climbed, our noses were overcome by the most aromatic smells and sensations. Some were familiar, like basil and mint, others completely new. "Sometimes, if I'm having a stressful day, I just come to this field and grab a bunch of lemon verbena and sit here and inhale and it boosts my brain into a better place," she chuckled. "It's cleansing."

"Try this," she said when we reached the patch. "It's French sorrel." It tasted strangely sour. "Like a tart apple, right? . . . And here's oregano, the Greek kind, which I like better than the Italian. It tastes about a million times better than the dried stuff. The CSA members often ask me, what's the difference between home and restaurant cooking? And I always tell them, it's the fresh herbs. They make all the difference." Chefs covet crops like radicchio and purslane, which have a bitter taste that home cooks find intimidating, but on a restaurant plate they add a nice touch of flavor. We moved through the herb garden, bending over, smelling, and tasting directly from the ground as we went. Jagoz was right—there is something soothing about the scent of fresh herbs.

We continued back toward the house, passing rows of more conventional herbs—parsley, cilantro, sage, mint—on our way. As we walked, we noticed bees and moths circling the field, dipping down here and there, collecting nectar. "I am trying to plant things that will attract pollinators for a longer period of the season. The fruits aren't blooming anymore, so we have things like clover because those can support whole colonies. When I moved here there weren't any pollinators around, but now they're coming." Their arrival is a testament to the ecologically harmonious and biodiverse community Jagoz is cultivating.

––––––––––

Jagoz's farm is an island in a sea of conventional agriculture. Every day is a reminder that she's going up against the system, not only as a vegan farmer but as a regenerative organic farmer too. When she moved onto her land, she had to get it tested. It was found to have extremely high levels of phosphorus, which, along with nitrogen and potassium, is one of the essential nutrients in healthy soil. But there can be too much of a good thing, and an abundance of phosphorus in soil is often a result of too much manure. Instead of spreading cow manure over ten thousand acres, for example, a farmer may have only a hundred, so it becomes overconcentrated and spoils the soil.

The Chesapeake Bay region is known for its dairy farms and chicken operations.[1] The mismanagement of animal waste leads to soil contamination. Nutrients seep through the soil into nearby waterways, causing environmental issues such as algae blooms that result in dead spots in the water.[2] Even though she in no way contributes to this toxicity, Jagoz is still required by the region to submit a "nutrient management plan" every year. The whole process is a cumbersome bureaucratic nightmare. She had to hire a nutrient management specialist to figure out how to navigate the system.

Dairy has been in decline for over a decade as consumers have been switching to alternatives made from soy, rice, nuts, and oats. The decline has led to a milk glut, leaving dairy farmers with excess milk that cannot be sold. No doubt dairy farmers are suffering, but the truth is that their operations are producing products that are not only unhealthy for many consumers (most of us are lactose intolerant), but polluting of the land as well. Yet dairy farmers, and those who grow corn and soy for cattle, still get government subsidies that ensure they stay in business. "I'm filling out all these forms, while there's this giant loophole for those who own cattle or horses. I don't see why they get the green light to pollute even though the dairy industry is in peril. It's such a colossal waste of land and of resources." Jagoz looked over the fields beyond her property wistfully and paused, seemingly lost in thought. "I want to prove that growing plants is better for our land, better for our health, and better for our communities. We *can* eat locally, if we just ate what was available seasonally, and we didn't expect to always get what we want."

Jagoz's vision for a more localized food system is realistic, and not only in places like California. A study out of the reputable Tufts Friedman School of Nutrition in Boston showed that if we were to drastically reduce our consumption of meat, it would substantially increase opportunities for rural regions like the one in which Jagoz lives and farms to grow their food for the cities nearby.[3] The problem now, as Jagoz explained, is how we choose to use the land. Immediately adjacent to her property are three fields growing soy and corn for animal feed. Other arable land is used to grow monocultures of wheat, soy, and corn for biofuels (crops used for energy) and for export to other countries (especially soy).

When Jagoz bought her property, she did so with an eye toward eventually acquiring the neighboring properties as well. To bring that to fruition, she began by asking her neighbors whether she could lease their land, but they all turned her down. Not because they were making a profit, but because the government subsidizes their crops and offers insurance regardless of whether their crops fail. There is no incentive for these farmers to change the status quo.

Let's step back for a moment and take this in: Farmers grow crops that have all sorts of damaging effects on local ecosystems. They sell those crops, unprofitably, to factory farms for animal feed that makes animals sick, in order to make products that in turn make us sick. Working together, both the government and subsidized farms produce food that ultimately serves no one except those who profit from the bottom line of meat, dairy, and egg sales. I don't know if you could invent a more broken food system if you tried.

Yet the odds are stacked against Jagoz and her farming vision, despite her best intentions and the benefits of her approach for animals and human health. If, for example, she wants to grow organic produce on her farm, the onus is on her to protect her plots from the conventional spray her neighbors use next door. She's had to plant numerous trees as a windbreak on the edges of her property, especially to the north, to ensure that her neighbors' spray doesn't affect her crops. If she gets "drift" from their pesticides on her farm, the consequences are hers to bear, not theirs.

She's also had to carve out several feet of land at each edge, where she cannot plant for fear of contamination. Last year, another organic grower she knows suffered the worst-case scenario—she was a victim of airplane spraying, a wasteful and imprecise way of spraying pesticides. On an especially windy day, the pesticides made it to her fields, and when her land was tested, they showed pesticide use. She lost her organic certification overnight. "It's not her fault, and she's devastated." Now she must wait three years before she can potentially regain her certification. That time frame is long enough for most farmers to lose their business, as many live on tiny margins.

I wondered, too, if Jagoz had to rely on some animal inputs to run her farm. I knew enough about conventional agriculture to know that fertilizers are almost always made of waste from factory farms. Given that these fertilizers contain high levels of phosphorus and nitrogen and contribute to soil runoff into local waterways, I wondered how Jagoz approached this issue not only as a regenerative farmer, but a vegan one too. She confirmed my suspicions: "We use mostly fish fertilizer, at this point, and some chicken-based fertilizer and bone meal"—made of leftover scraps from slaughtered animals. "I don't like using it, but I don't know what else to do. I know another vegan farmer in south Maryland who's been doing organic farming for thirty years, and he has high-quality crops. I told him, I'm vegan too, how did you fix the fertilizer problem? And he chuckled at me, like 'Oh, honey,'" implying the impracticality of her desire to do away with conventional agriculture altogether.

For a while, Jagoz became obsessed with finding a healthful vegan alternative to animal-based fertilizer, but she could not find a way out of the system. "Besides being expensive, vegan fertilizers are often made of GMO soy, so that's not organic, or the alternative stuff is out of stock. And I have all this equipment that's made for pelletized fertilizer, so even if you get the stuff that's not conventional, it's impossible to spread it around at scale." With animal farms enjoying market dominance and government subsidies, incentives to create alternative fertilizers are virtually nonexistent.

The other thing on my mind was pests. How does she protect her produce against pests in a way that avoids harming wild animals? "We have a pest management system," she says. "We must, otherwise they'll ruin our crops. We do have to use some organic sprays, but we try to use as much equipment and organic means of pest control as possible." One method is using covers for the rows of produce, which also keep the seedlings a few degrees warmer and protected from frost. Handpicking caterpillars, though, is unrealistic at scale, and minimal spraying of organic spray becomes inevitable.

I wondered whether Jagoz believed that fully "veganic" farming—farming without the use of any animal inputs—is possible at all. "I mean, it's practical to use animals in farming. If you fence them in, they will not only trim your grass and stomp out weeds, but they'll also give you your fertilizer. Personally," she continued, "I think using horsepower on a farm makes sense, especially to reduce tractor use. There's a reason our agricultural system was built upon having animals. Many people wouldn't consider that vegan farming, but I do." The real problem with using animals in a holistic system is that they aren't rotated on the land nearly enough to justify the argument that they add value to the soil. "It's a delicate balance, and so it takes a lot of land to keep animals on happy grass."

Still, farming without animal inputs remains her dream. "My mission is to change the landscape of agriculture in the mid-Atlantic because it's so messed up. You know, in the small-scale ag world, there's a lot of cynicism, not only about Silicon Valley and its plant-based proteins, but also about whether veganism is possible given the agricultural system we have. They say, you know, when you get to the real world, you need animals as part of the system. But I think there's a way of working with animals without eating them or extracting from them."

If Jagoz could afford it, she would use the properties around her land to plant cover crops and make her own compost as fertilizer. She told me there's a farm in Pennsylvania that has perfected this model. "They have two hundred acres, but they only grow vegetables on fifty, and the rest they use to make fertilizer. That farmer isn't vegan, but he's doing it for ethical reasons. He doesn't want to buy product from a sick industry to feed his healthy plants. I'm looking toward solutions like that, but I need more land."

It's a common refrain in the food world that one of the biggest hurdles for young farmers, if not *the* biggest, is access to land. Especially for those who have traditionally had no access, there are rarely legacy plans in place to pass off land from older to younger farmers. Farmers also compete with inefficient uses of potentially arable land—golf courses, football fields, and parking lots, all of which drive Jagoz mad—"We could be growing food on those golf courses!" Jagoz's strategy for obtaining land at the start was to barter parcel by parcel in exchange for a CSA share. But it helped a lot that her parents had been living in the same community for thirty years. That's not the case for many aspiring farmers, especially minority farmers.

Imagine if we could replace inefficient uses of land with fields of polycropped lentils, beans, and nuts that could feed a growing world population, allowing people to eat far more locally, not to mention healthfully and sustainably. Then, maybe, farming would be an economically viable and fulfilling career option, with a restored sense of pride that writers such as the legendary farmer and writer Wendell Berry show has been lost. One of Jagoz's personal heroes is the renowned organic farmer Eliot Coleman, who once said, "The only truly dependable production technologies are those that are sustainable over the long term." Coleman authored the bible of organic agriculture—*The New Organic Grower*.[4] Jagoz read everything he wrote and, step by step, followed his instructions for how to set up an operational organic farm.

The farming Jagoz is practicing is in alignment with the "regenerative agriculture" model I was reading about back in Berkeley, and I wondered what she thought of the term. "I mean, like any buzzword, it's problematic when people can just say, Oh, I'm 'sustainable' or 'regenerative.' What that means on the ground varies widely farm to farm. I haven't seen any convincing or consistent definition. But I guess to me, it means paying attention to your land, working with the land. If your soil pH is 7.5 (alkaline), don't plant blueberries, because they need a lower pH (acidic). I mean, you could try to plant blueberries, but then you'd have to put in a lot of effort and a lot of inputs and that's kind of the opposite of saying 'Let me play to my strengths.' I try to combine my talents with the needs of my market to create a financially viable business. Farming is always a negotiation between your ideals and the reality on the ground."

As an organic farmer with a diversified crop, Jagoz must constantly adjust her decisions and what she works on each day in response to the weather. Too hot, too cold, too dry, too wet—these conditions dictate her entire life. That's something farmers growing monoculture (single-crop) fields with chemical fertilizer, genetically modified crops, and pesticides never have to worry about. And if they do lose a crop, they have government protection through subsidies and insurance. It's not that their lives are easy, because often they aren't making a profit, but compared to all the "cognitive labor" Jagoz does every day, the "farming" they do is far less dynamic, complex, and, frankly, challenging.

Jagoz is constantly negotiating between what needs to be done now, in the short term, versus her ambitions for the farm on the horizon. For instance, should she plant cash crops that will make money next season, or a cover crop like buckwheat or alfalfa that can't be harvested but will "add value" to the soil quality over the long term? If she wants to be profitable, she should choose the former. If she wants her farm to be sustainable, she must choose the latter. Most of the time, she doesn't have much choice since she just needs to make money to pay her workers and feed her family.

The pas de deux between a farmer and her land is a dance most of us aren't cognizant of at all. As consumers we want cherry tomatoes all summer, but we may not realize that for organic farmers in the mid-Atlantic region, cherry tomatoes are hard to grow. Unless you're lucky enough to live on the coast of California, the options for buying organic, locally grown crops year around are limited. Even in the Bay Area, where I stick to mostly what's available at the farmers market, cherry tomatoes are around for only a few weeks in the summertime. If only a few more of us would accept the ecological realities of where we live—how to cook kohlrabi rather than always expecting broccolini to be available, for example—we could learn to eat well while supporting the sustainable regenerative practices of farmers like Jagoz.

————

After we toured her fields, Jagoz invited Douglas and me in for a wholesome farmer's meal made from the foods she sells to her CSA members. She grabbed a few handfuls of fresh maitake mushrooms from her fungi vendor (I only learned what these are when I moved to California, and they're probably the most delicious mushrooms I have ever tried), as well as a loaf of sourdough bread from a local bakery. The kitchen, like the rest of the house, is spacious, with a sitting area to one side and French doors leading off to the main room, painted green and full of plants, almost like a conservatory, which I recognized from our video calls.

Jagoz placed a big cast iron pan on the stovetop, heating up some olive oil and garlic. When they began to sizzle, she threw in the maitake mushrooms along with some tamari, and within minutes, the whole kitchen was filled with a savory umami aroma, making my stomach grumble. Jagoz handed me a few vegetables from her farm—mixed lettuces, radicchio, green bell peppers, carrots, white turnips, and mint. As I cut these up and dressed them with fresh lemon juice and balsamic vinegar, the salad came to life. Then Jagoz took out some of the sauerkraut and jalapeños she'd pickled herself, and asked Douglas to toast the bread. When everything was ready, we sat down at the dining room table, looking out the picture window onto the fields. We dug into the meal, weighing down the generous sourdough slices with sautéed mushrooms, sauerkraut, and pickled jalapeños, and taking satisfying bites in between of the crunchy freshness of the salad.

Over lunch, Jagoz told us more stories about life on the farm, and I asked her about the most common questions she receives. "'What do you do all winter?'" she answered, with a slight smirk. "It's a valid question, but I find it funny because people grossly underestimate what it takes to be a farmer. They minimize what it takes to be a business owner on top of growing food. What do I do? Well, I've got a year of paperwork to catch up on, all my accounting that I didn't have time to do while working eighteen-hour days, the marketing and logistics to figure out how to sell my produce, and all the equipment I need to fix. So, I do a lot." She used to work on weekends but realized after a few years that it wasn't sustainable, especially as a single parent with two children. Now she tries to take one day off a week to be with her family.

The other question she gets often, especially from journalists, is "How do we make farming sexy?" "I always laugh at that question. It's like, well, how about making it a viable career option, with benefits and time off? The interest is there, I think, but people need health insurance and a healthy work-life balance. Farming can take over your life, and because you're far from the city, it's not the kind of thing a lot of young people want to do." Thankfully, she received a seed grant from the USDA that will help her hire two full-time staff members for the next two years, a huge boon for her business, in which labor is probably the biggest hurdle to business growth.

I found Jagoz's dedication incredibly inspiring. Each day, she wakes before dawn to farm because she's trying to build a better food system, not only for her children, but for us all. We are about the same age, and she too became vegan in her early twenties. But while we both care deeply about building a better food system, my path has mostly been confined to the realm of ideas. Jagoz's path has been to get her hands dirty, literally, and I found myself admiring her entrepreneurial, action-oriented energy.

On our way out, I spotted a framed poster by the door that captured Jagoz's essence: a drawing of a worker bee with the caption "Things may come to those who wait, but only the things left by those who *hustle*."

———————

Our last stop in D.C. before returning home was at Ellē, a high-end restaurant in the trendy Mount Pleasant neighborhood recommended to us by Jagoz as a place that sources from her farm. We don't eat out often, but when we do we enjoy the farm-to-table creativity of chefs who turn boxes of fresh produce into culinary delights. That week, Jagoz had sold the restaurant fresh ginger and turmeric, but she often sells many other vegetables. We called ahead to request a vegan tasting menu, and when we arrived, we decided to splurge.

The first course was a homemade seitan with creamy avocado sauce, which tasted wonderfully umami and salty. Then came a course of beets in a hazelnut cream sauce, and a pear salad with radicchio (just as Jagoz had said) and spring greens. The main course was a satisfyingly thick pasta with local mushrooms and a crunchy vegan bacon on top. But it was the final plate that turned out to be the pièce de resistance: a spaghetti squash tartine on sourdough bread with truffle gratings. We had recently watched the wonderful *Truffle Hunters* documentary and were excited to try the mythical fungi for the first time. As we marveled at the dinner I wondered what would happen if all of us ate more like Jagoz wished—filling our plates with fruits, vegetables, legumes, and whole grains, as seasonally and locally as possible. What kind of benefits, individually and collectively, could such a diet bring? Not only on our environment, but for ourselves?

Chapter Eight

You Are What You Eat

Like a lost jewel that takes greater effort to find than it does to keep in the first instance, good health, once it is lost, costs much time and effort to regain.

—Mahatma Gandhi

In 1982, a renowned biochemist at Cornell University named T. Colin Campbell was called upon to present his research at the National Institutes of Health. Dr. Campbell's work is controversial. Not for lack of scientific soundness, but because its conclusions fly in the face of conventional nutritional wisdom. His research shows that consuming animal protein increases the incidence of cancer. Dr. Campbell was himself surprised by the results, as he grew up on a dairy farm and always believed milk to be "nature's perfect food."[1] He knew that advocating for a vegetarian diet (he hadn't even heard of the word "vegan" at that time) would raise eyebrows, so he had to come up with a different way to describe it. As he told the New York Times almost four decades later, "I wanted to emphasize that my work and ideas were coming totally from science and not any sort of ethical or philosophical consideration."[2]

Dr. Campbell thought carefully about how he could talk about the dietary patterns he had in mind: animal-free, low in fat, high in fiber, and made up of ingredients like starches, legumes, fruits, and vegetables, rather than substitutes or alternatives popular among vegetarians at the time. As he explains on the website of the T. Colin Campbell Center for Nutrition Studies, "My solution was to choose 'plant-based' for lack of a better word. I also thought that the idea had to rest on good solid science, if it were to survive. Still today, I avoid the 'V' words because most vegetarians consume too much processed food and total fat. I added 'whole' to my 'plant-based' nomenclature a little later, to avoid the idea that isolated nutrients (as in supplements) and/or plant food fragments (refined carbohydrates like sugar and white flour) conveyed health. My considerable experience in court testifying to the inappropriate use of nutrient supplements compelled me to add the word 'whole' as in 'whole food, plant-based.' "[3]

The year after he presented to the panel, Dr. Campbell began an ambitious study with collaborators Dr. Junshi Chen of the Chinese Institute of Nutrition and Food Hygiene and Professor Richard Peto of the University of Oxford. The idea was to track the eating habits of sixty-five hundred Chinese people across many provinces and look specifically at the link between diet and cancer, but eventually other diseases including heart, metabolic, and infectious diseases. The setting was ideal, since rural Chinese ate nearly entirely plant-based diets, while their urban counterparts ate more animal protein (though still far less than in Western countries).

In the first wave of the study (1983–84), the researchers selected sixty-five rural counties, within which two villages were selected, with fifty families in each randomly chosen to participate. One adult from each household (half men and half women) provided blood, urine, and food samples, as well a questionnaire and diet diaries for three consecutive days.[4] In the second wave of the study, six years later (1989–90), the same counties and individuals were surveyed, and twenty new counties and twenty additional families per county were added from mainland China and Taiwan, for a total of 10,200 adults and their families. This time, socioeconomic data was collected for all participants.[5]

No study of this scale and magnitude had ever been done before, and in 1990, when the *New York Times* wrote about the initial results, they dubbed it the "Grand Prix" of epidemiology.[6] The article opens with, "Early findings from the most comprehensive large study ever undertaken of the relationship between diet and the risk of developing disease are challenging much of American dietary dogma. The study, being conducted in China, paints a bold portrait of a plant-based eating plan that is more likely to promote health than disease." Indeed, Dr. Campbell and his colleagues found that the Chinese ate only a third of the protein of the average American, and far less of it was of animal origin. In fact, the Chinese who ate the most protein, especially from animals (only richer families who could afford it), had the highest rates of chronic disease, just like Westerners.

Less protein, not more? Hadn't we been worrying about getting *enough* protein all this time? In fact, the study suggested that *more* protein is harmful. In the last thirty years, further research has confirmed that animal protein is harmful for our health, no matter if it's organic or grass-fed. One study of more than four hundred thousand subjects found that swapping just 3 percent of calories from animal protein for plant protein lowered the risk of death by 10 percent over a sixteen-year period,[7] and another confirmed that eating saturated fat from a plant rather than an animal led to a longer life span.[8] As long as you eat a variety of plants—including grains, legumes, fruits, and vegetables—you will acquire all of the essential amino acids your body requires.[9] In fact, when vegans eat a healthful plant-rich diet, they have far higher intakes of many essential vitamins, as well as fiber, folate, magnesium, and iron.[10]

In terms of macronutrient ratios—of carbohydrates, fats, and protein—research suggests that ideally, no more than 10 to 15 percent of our calories should be protein, and from as few animal sources as possible.[11] These finding fly completely in the face of the Dietary Guidelines for Americans, which for years promoted the idea that protein should make up 30 percent of our calories. As Dr. Campbell concluded back in the '90s, "We're basically a vegetarian species and should be eating a wide variety of plant foods and minimizing our intake of animal foods."[12]

In 2005, Dr. Campbell published *The China Study* with his son Thomas M. Campbell, detailing the results of the study along with additional research for a popular audience. Initially not widely known, the book became a bestseller through word of mouth and was featured prominently in the film *Forks over Knives*, which follows his story alongside that of other pioneering doctors advocating for the plant-based way of life, including Dr. Caldwell Esselstyn, Dr. John McDougall, Dr. Michael Klaper, and Dr. Alan Goldhammer.

Dr. Esselstyn's clinical work famously showed that putting critically ill heart patients on a low-fat whole foods plant-based diet could not only stall but potentially reverse the progression of chronic disease, eliminating ailments such as heart disease and diabetes, among the top causes of morbidity in the Western world.[13] In fact, this type of diet is consistently shown to be healthier than even other well-known and widely promoted diets, including the Mediterranean diet.[14] What's beneficial about a Mediterranean diet isn't only what it contains—far more whole vegetables, fruits, grains, legumes, nuts, and seeds than in a typical American diet—but what it largely doesn't: butter, eggs, meat, and processed foods.[15]

Studies on the link between dairy and cancer have been mixed, some suggesting that it's protective and others suggesting the opposite. Dr. Walter Willett, a prominent researcher at the Harvard T. H. Chan School of Public Health, has shown that the contradictory findings may be linked in part to context—in places where people are malnourished, dairy provides essential nutrients (protein, calcium, and vitamin D)[16] that people can't otherwise easily obtain. But in places where people don't need dairy to survive, it is harmful, especially as it contains saturated fat, cholesterol, and lactose, which is not easily digestible by most people (especially minority individuals, but even those with European ancestry).[17]

Since *The China Study* came out, the benefits of a healthful plant-based lifestyle have been published in top medical journals all around the world. A comprehensive study in *JAMA* (*Journal of the American Medical Association*) found that dietary factors are the leading cause of death from the top killers in our society: heart disease, stroke, and type 2 diabetes.[18] In 2017, *The Lancet*, a prestigious international medical journal, published results from the Global Burden of Disease Study. This is the largest and most comprehensive study ever conducted on premature deaths (across 204 countries). Its conclusion? That lifestyle factors are now the primary cause of half of early deaths and, perhaps surprisingly, an unhealthful diet is even worse for health than smoking or lack of exercise.[19] Just imagine what would happen if there were suddenly a large-scale shift toward healthier life-styles—the economic, social, and political impact is hard to fathom.[20]

Despite the significance of these results, today's medical students still get only a few hours of nutritional education. My sister Galina, who earned her degree at Harvard Medical School, told me that her nutritional instruction amounted to groups of medical students being assigned different diets to examine and report back to the class a couple of hours later, and that's the norm in most medical school programs.[21] As Dr. Esselstyn told me a few years ago at PlantStock (a play on Woodstock), a plant-based convention: "It's still the Dark Ages in medical schools. Chronic illness can be avoided with whole foods plant-based nutrition but there's a lot of money involved in bypasses and cardiac stents and statin drugs. The cause of disease is not genetic, it's habitual."

———

These days, the idea of "lifestyle medicine"[22] is in vogue—everywhere you look, it seems that people are waking up the idea that diet, exercise, sleep habits, and stress management are directly related to disease. Products like biometric trackers and services like personal trainers are all the rage. Various flavors of the "clean eating" trend have promoted products as varied as celery juice, bone broth, and coconut oil. But it wasn't always this way.

Dr. Dean Ornish knows this all too well. Dr. Ornish is famous for helping Bill Clinton slim down before his daughter's wedding on a low-fat whole foods plant-based diet. But it took him a long time, and lots of askance looks and raised eyebrows, to prove that diet and lifestyle were important factors in shaping not only the longevity but the quality of our lives. Dr. Ornish's inspiration to bring meaning to the lives of others comes from knowing what it's like to lose it.

From a well-to-do family, Dr. Ornish always felt pressure to compete academically. As a freshman at Rice University in Houston, Texas, his battle with impostor syndrome became so severe that he started drinking and taking tranquilizers to cope, but it wasn't helping. The existential angst became so profound that he seriously contemplated suicide, even imagining throwing himself off a big oil derrick near the end zone of the college football field. "I had a spiritual vision," he told me when we met a few years ago at his office in Sausalito, just north of the Golden Gate Bridge in San Francisco, "that nothing can bring lasting happiness, and so I wondered, what's the point of living?"

The stress was so great that the young Dr. Ornish suffered a severe case of mononucleosis and was sent home to Dallas to recuperate. While he was there, his parents hosted a cocktail party for a swami with whom his older sister had been studying in India. Swami Satchidananda looked exactly, as Dr. Ornish puts it, "like Central Casting's idea of a swami—long white beard, peaceful eyes, long saffron robe." The swami's own master was Swami Sivananda, himself a physician and renowned founder of the Divine Life Society, an ashram in Rishikesh, India, and the mentor of my own teacher when I began studying in Toronto, Canada. Sivananda officially ordained Satchidananda in 1949, after which he began to travel and spread his teachings.

The swami had a profound impact on the soon-to-be doctor. "They say that when a student is ready, a teacher comes. I had figured out that nothing can bring lasting happiness, which led me to become suicidally depressed, but he was teaching the same thing, yet he was glowing. So, I was like, what am I missing here?" When Dr. Ornish asked the swami whether he was a Hindu, the guru punned, "No, I'm an Undo." His central philosophy was that peace comes not from doing but from undoing, not from getting but from letting go. The purpose of all spiritual practices, he believed, is to stop disturbing what you already have—the Buddhist idea of the "whole" within.[23]

The swami became a mentor to the doctor, leaving a profound imprint on his life and ultimately, on his career in medicine. Among the swami's teachings was an emphasis on a simple vegetarian diet (which inspired the young doctor to give up meat in 1972), stress reduction through yoga and meditation, and living in harmony with nature. Although he spoke highly of the benefits of Western medicine, he felt they should be integrated with Eastern models of homeopathy and naturopathy as well. One of the central tenets of the philosophy was the idea that our natural state is to be at ease, and that it is only when we disturb this natural state through habits like smoking, drinking, drug use, unhealthy foods, stress, and a sedentary lifestyle that we become "*dis*-eased."

After finishing his undergraduate degree at the University of Texas at Austin (he had dropped out of Rice during his depression), Dr. Ornish went on to earn his medical degree at Baylor College of Medicine in Houston in 1980. While there, he put the swami's teachings into practice. He asked his supervisor for referrals to his patients so he could launch a study looking at the effects of yoga, stress reduction, and a vegetarian diet on patients with heart disease. He was only a second-year medical student at the time, and such requests were unheard of, especially on the terrain of Dr. Michael DeBakey, the inventor of the cardiac bypass procedure. Although the procedure saved some lives, it also meant that the doctors were "literally and figuratively bypassing the problem," as Dr. Ornish put it. "We'd cut people open, but then they'd go home and eat junk food and not manage stress or exercise and keep smoking and drinking."

Dr. Ornish wondered if there was another way, and he eventually managed to get approval for a pilot program with ten people—seven men and three women—who agreed to live in a hotel for free for one month. The participants ate low-fat vegetarian meals and Dr. Ornish lectured and taught yoga daily. By the end of the month, they found an impressive 91 percent reduction in angina and chest pain and significantly improved blood flow. When Dr. Ornish finished medical school, he became a clinical fellow at Harvard Medical School, but he found the pioneering spirit of Texas lacking in the Boston establishment medical culture. "I realized I could stay there and work in someone else's lab for a decade, and only then would I be able to do my own studies, so I left."

He accepted a teaching position at the University of California School of Medicine in San Francisco and founded a nonprofit, the Preventive Medicine Research Institute (PMRI). Since 1984, it has run clinical trials looking at whether lifestyle choices can be as powerful as, or even in some cases more powerful than, treating disease with conventional medical interventions. Their first study was the Lifestyle Heart Trial, a randomized controlled trial in which participants limited their dietary fat intake to only 10 percent of calories (mostly by cutting out high-fat animal products and processed foods) as well doing yoga, meditating, exercising moderately, and participating in a support group.

The landmark study, published in *JAMA*, showed that even severe heart disease can be reversed by the Ornish Program after only a month.[24] Episodes of chest pain decreased by 91 percent after only a few weeks. In a five-year follow-up, there was even more reversal of coronary artery blockages than after one year, 2.5 times fewer cardiac events, and a 300 percent improvement in blood flow to the heart.[25] Virtually all patients were able to stop or reverse their heart disease after five years, a finding that shocked many cardiologists when it was published in *The Lancet*, putting Dr. Ornish and his program on the medical map.

In 2005, Dr. Ornish and his colleagues moved on to prostate cancer, similarly showing, for the first time, that the progression of early-stage prostate cancer can be halted and even reversed by the Ornish program. In 2008, they showed that after only three months, patients' actual genes changed: the ones that enhance health turned on, and the ones that promote disease turned off.[26] In fact, other work has clearly shown that diet and lifestyle may alter gene expression,[27] but further work needs to be done to understand how, precisely, genes interact with lifestyle factors.[28]

The institute published another study in the journal *Lancet Oncology* in collaboration with Dr. Elizabeth Blackburn of UCSF School of Medicine, who won a Nobel Prize in Medicine for her discovery of telomeres in 2009.[29] Telomeres are the structures at the ends of chromosomes that keep our DNA from unraveling (like the aglets on the tips of shoelaces). Shorter telomeres mean a shorter lifespan. Dr. Ornish and his colleagues showed that lifestyle interventions can lengthen telomeres, slowing down the unraveling process.[30] These results show us that while genes may be hereditary, diets too are passed down in families, and they contribute a lot more to our health than we give them credit for.

Dr. Ornish began setting up clinics around the country to implement his program. But even as it began to change lives for the better, he ran into a major roadblock: medical insurance. For the program to be practical, it needed to be covered by Medicare. If it wasn't reimbursed, it wouldn't have much effect in practice. Easy, he thought, it would take a few months. But when Dr. Ornish first met with the director of Medicare in 1993, he was told, "If we cover this, anyone with a crystal and a pyramid will want us to pay for what they do."

In the end, the process to get the Ornish program approved by Medicare turned out to take sixteen years. It required comprehensive review by leading physicians and scientists, many of them skeptical of a lifestyle-based approach, given their backgrounds in conventional medicine, which is all about pills and procedures. One of the requirements was a letter from the National Institutes of Health certifying that the program was safe. "I thought, you must be joking," says Dr. Ornish. "You mean, I need a letter to certify that it's safe to walk, meditate, eat well, quit smoking, and love more?" Ironically, years later, trials showed that cardiac bypasses were largely ineffective, and results were mostly due to placebo effects.

Eventually, the Centers for Medicare and Medicaid Services (CMS) approved Dr. Ornish's program on August 12, 2010.[31] They created a whole new benefit category called "intensive cardiac rehabilitation" (ICR) and began providing Medicare coverage for "Dr. Dean Ornish's Program for

Reversing Heart Disease," which included 72 hours of interventions for those who experienced heart attacks, chest pain, heart valve repair, bypasses, or stents. Not only was this the first integrative medicine program to be covered by medical insurance, but perhaps even more amazingly, it had bipartisan support, including from President Bill Clinton and Newt Gingrich, Speaker of the House. For once, the Democrats and Republicans agreed on something.

Describing the program in a recent op-ed in the *New York Times* called "The Myth of High-Protein Diets,"[32] Dr. Ornish wrote: "An optimal diet for preventing disease is a whole foods, plant-based diet that is naturally low in animal protein, harmful fats, and refined carbohydrates. What that means in practice is little or no red meat; mostly vegetables, fruits, whole grains, legumes, and soy products in their natural forms; very few simple and refined carbohydrates such as sugar and white flour; and sufficient 'good fats' such as fish oil or flax oil, seeds, and nuts. A healthful diet should be low in 'bad fats,' meaning trans fats, saturated fats, and hydrogenated fats. Finally, we need more quality and less quantity."

Of course, not everyone is on board with the Ornish Lifestyle Program. One often-cited criticism is a piece in the *Scientific American* by the science journalist Melinda Wenner Moyer in response to Dr. Ornish's *New York Times* op-ed. Moyer identified what she perceives as a vilification of dietary fat (in the Ornish program, dietary fat accounts for a mere 10 percent of calories, much lower than the 30 percent recommended by the American Heart Association). She also criticized the lifestyle program for incorporating other components including smoking and drinking cessation, moderate exercise, stress reduction through yoga and meditation, and support groups, arguing that these components make it unclear whether diet alone is impactful.

Part of the problem with Moyer's first point is that it's not only the amount of fat in a diet, but also the *type*. It's been shown repeatedly not only by Dr. Ornish but by others that animal-derived fat is more harmful than plant-based fat. In 2012, a huge study from the Harvard School of Public Health of more than 37,000 men and women showed that red meat consumption is associated with an overall increased risk of death, and that a portion of these deaths can be prevented simply by reducing animal consumption significantly.[33] The same is true for cardiovascular disease, cancer, and type 2 diabetes, among other preventable illnesses.

What mechanisms account for the harms of a high-fat, high-protein diet? It appears that besides raising cholesterol levels, diets high in animal products cause arterial blockages, elevate levels of free fatty acids and insulin, lower the production of endothelial progenitor cells (which keep arteries clean), and increase the production of IGF-1, an insulin-like growth hormone that causes chronic inflammation, as well as Neu5Gc, a tumor-forming sugar that likely plays a role in promoting cancer growth.

The bottom line, as Dr. Ornish puts it, is simple: "The only diet that has been scientifically proven to reverse heart disease, to slow, stop, or reverse early-stage prostate cancer, and to reverse aging by lengthening telomeres is a whole-foods plant-based diet low in both fat and refined carbohydrates."[34] Sure, the other components of the program are helpful on their own, but even more so in concert with each other. Moyer's criticism obscures the fact that despite disagreements at the margins, nutritional science is coming to a clear consensus around the optimal diet. As the American Dietetic Association summarized back in 2009: "It is the position of the American Dietetic Association that appropriately planned vegetarian diets, including total vegetarian or vegan diets, are healthful, nutritionally adequate, and may provide health benefits in the prevention and treatment of certain diseases."[35]

There is a unifying thesis to Dr. Ornish's work, and it is this: All diseases are variations on a theme. Under the hood, they share the same underlying biological mechanisms. Chronic inflammation, problems in the microbiome, telomeres and gene expression, oxidative stress, impaired immune function, and overstimulation of the sympathetic nervous system are all influenced by what we eat, how much we exercise, whether we manage our stress, and whether our lives are filled with intimacy and connection. That's why the same person will often have multiple diseases (called comorbidities)—obesity, for example, often goes hand in hand with high blood pressure, high cholesterol, and pre-diabetes. It turns out that when people implement healthier lifestyle behaviors, they get better overall, which suggests these factors are intimately interconnected.[36]

In many ways, this kind of advice flies in the face of the recent trend toward personalized medicine, which says that there is too much diversity in the human population for a one-size-fits-all approach. True, there is genetic diversity among individuals, and even whole populations, with some being able to digest the lactose in dairy products and gluten in wheat products better than others. But, as Dr. Ornish once wrote to President Bill Clinton: "Our genes are a predisposition, but our genes are not our fate. You're genetically predisposed to having heart disease because it runs in your family, but that just means that you need to make bigger changes to prevent or reverse it than someone else might. Our DNA is not our destiny."[37]

Given how long it has taken Dr. Ornish to convince the public of the power of diet (as well as exercise, social connection, and stress-reducing activities), I wondered what gives him the faith to keep promoting lifestyle medicine. "That's a good question," he answered. "No one's asked me that before. I think it's because when I made the decision not to kill myself, it gave me the courage to try anything and without fear. I made a vow that I would live a messy life. I would make mistakes, but I would live it. Everything I've done since then was something others thought was impossible." To this day, spirituality imbues not only his life, but also his medical practice, and Dr. Ornish has realized that fear isn't a good motivator because it's not sustainable. Instead, he lives from a place of joy, and he advises his patients to do the same.

———

In 2018, Dr. Ornish embarked on his most ambitious quest yet: to show that lifestyle interventions can help prevent, even reverse, not only illnesses of the body, but of the mind as well. His latest ongoing study is with Alzheimer's patients, a new frontier of lifestyle medicine. According to the Alzheimer's Association, more than six million Americans are currently living with Alzheimer's disease, and a third of seniors have Alzheimer's or other forms of dementia at the time of death.[38] As alarming as these statistics are, they are likely underreporting the true prevalence of dementia because people think that fading memory (such as misplacing keys or mixing up grandchildren's names) is a normal part of the aging process. These diseases cost the nation $355 billion annually, and the cost is estimated to reach over a trillion dollars by 2050.

Like many people, I assumed that Alzheimer's disease was mostly a genetic roll of the dice, and that if you had the "bad" genes, there wasn't that much you could do about it. Yet only about 3 percent of Alzheimer's disease cases are determined by genes.[39] Neurologists now estimate that about 90 percent of Alzheimer's disease is preventable through a healthy lifestyle, especially diet, and the same is true of other forms of dementia.[40] Like many people, I never quite made the connection that diseases of the mind are linked to diseases of the body. It's an assumption typical in the Western model of medicine, which focuses on individual parts rather than the system as a whole.

Yet when you think about it, if we know that a high-fat, low-carb diet affects one organ—the heart—why not also the brain?[41] One study measured the cholesterol levels of nearly ten thousand people between 1964 and 1973, and then followed them for forty years to find that high cholesterol in midlife increased the chance of developing Alzheimer's later on by 57 percent and dementia by 26 percent.[42] Other studies have shown that those who eat a plant-based diet have less risk of cognitive impairment in later life.[43] Just as blood vessels supply oxygen to the heart, they supply it also to the vital tissues in our brain. Alzheimer's is, in essence, the "heart disease of the brain."[44]

For many people, a diagnosis of Alzheimer's is akin to a death sentence, as people gradually lose their sense of self. As Dr. Ornish says, "When you lose your memories, you lose everything." That's why he and colleagues from PMRI are collaborating with the University of California, San Francisco School of Medicine, the Harvard Medical School / Massachusetts General Hospital (MGH) in Boston, the Lou Ruvo Center for Brain Health at the Cleveland Clinic in Las Vegas, and the University of California, San Diego, to conduct the first randomized controlled trial of whether early-stage Alzheimer's can be slowed through lifestyle changes.

The key outcome the team is interested in is cognitive function, but they are also looking at changes in telomere length at Dr. Elizabeth Blackburn's lab at UCSF, changes in the microbiome at Dr. Rob Knight's Center for Microbiome Innovation at UCSD, Dr. Rudy Tanzi's genetics and aging lab at Harvard University, Dr. Steven Arnold's neurology lab at MGH, and Dr. David Sinclair's aging lab at Harvard Medical School. The goal of the study is to understand the precise mechanisms by which lifestyle changes affect the progression of Alzheimer's disease.

In September 2018, one hundred patients living in San Francisco, San Diego, Boston, and Las Vegas were randomly assigned to two groups. Both groups were tested at baseline. Then one group retested after twenty weeks on the lifestyle medicine program, while the control group was told not to change any habits. After the first group was tested, the second group also began receiving the treatment ("crossing over" into the treatment group) and were retested as well at the halfway point (so as not to deny the control group the benefits if in fact the program proved effective). After a total of forty weeks, both groups were retested and compared.

Throughout the process, all meals (twenty-one meals a week) were provided free of charge to patients as well as their spouses or caregivers. Patients were also trained in stress management and exercise and engaged in a support group three days a week for four hours. At the onset of the coronavirus pandemic in March 2020, all of these activities moved onto Zoom, and meals were shipped directly to patients' homes, but the program continued virtually.

When I first met Dr. Ornish in person, I had a chance to meet some of the participants in the program while they were having lunch on the ground floor of PMRI. I hadn't spent time with anyone with Alzheimer's before, and I didn't know what to expect. As we all sat down with our plant-based soup, steamed veggies, and stew, I noticed that some had a harder time formulating sentences than others, over-articulating certain words or stalling between them. As Dr. Ornish later explained in his office, "Alzheimer's is a profoundly isolating experience. You're told there's nothing you can do. We'll be taking away your driver's license and you better get your affairs in order. It's a kind of emotional and spiritual pain, a loss of hope. That sense of hopelessness leads to depression, and I know from my own experience that it can lead you to unspeakable places."

At the time of this writing, the results of the study have not yet been published (the study should be complete by the end of 2023), but the early findings appear promising. Dr. Ornish is hopeful, believing that we are at a turning point with Alzheimer's just as we have been with coronary heart disease and cancer. Currently, there is no drug on the market that offers a truly promising cure for Alzheimer's. If lifestyle interventions can make a difference, the implications are profound. "Of course, we don't know if it will work," Dr. Ornish told me, "but imagine that it does. How much hope would that give millions of Americans? Not only those diagnosed with this fate, but all of those who love and care for them?" As he likes to say about lifestyle medicine: "What you gain is so much more than what you give up."

In June 2021, I had the chance to ask some of those in the study directly about their experiences. Dr. Ornish invited me to join a virtual support group for a week, which he led. At the start, he asked each patient how they were feeling, helped them connect with the loved ones present with them and, as it happened the week I joined, experience the therapeutic power of music. At one point, the entire group joined in singing the classic Eagles song "Desperado"—some could remember the lyrics better than others, but all laughed, cried, and bonded with one another. As Dr. Ornish repeated to the group multiple times, "Anything that brings us closer together and away from isolation and loneliness heals us."

Over the years, many have raised eyebrows at Dr. Ornish's boldness, skeptical that lifestyle interventions alone can address many of the most pressing chronic diseases faced by Western populations. But his work has repeatedly shown the power of behavioral interventions not only to cure disease but to lead to a more satisfying and meaningful life, just like the one gifted to him by his spiritual teacher. His work clearly shows that Hippocrates's precept "Let food be thy medicine" is as true today as ever before.

Chapter Nine

Cult to Cool

Lately as plant-based eating has blossomed and gained followers, influential vegans are laboring to supplant its dowdy, spartan image with a new look: glamorous, prosperous, sexy, and epidermally beaming with health.

—*New York Times*

I 'm going to have the alfalfa sprouts and mashed yeast." That's the unappetizing order made by Alvy Singer (Woody Allen) at a vegetarian restaurant in Los Angeles in the 1977 cult classic film *Annie Hall*. The restaurant, with its brown-and-green color scheme, patio furniture, and veggie menu, was in fact a real place. The Source opened on April Fool's Day in 1969 on Sunset Strip. Above the wide patio, a towering round sign loomed. The circle contained a pyramid with an eye at its center. The Eye of Providence is found on the back of the American dollar bill, symbolizing the coming of a new world order. The two mottoes surrounding the circle read: *Annuit coeptis* ("Providence favors our undertakings") and *Novus ordo seclorum* ("New order of the ages"). Inside the restaurant were a brick fireplace decorated with multicolored candles, stained-glass windows, and a mural of a man encased inside a pentagram.

The Source was one of the first vegetarian restaurants in the country. The menu offered what we now think of as "hippie food": vegetable juices, fruit smoothies, herbal teas, brown rice, nut and seed bars, carob chocolate, avocado, nutritional yeast, and the infamous alfalfa sprouts. The restaurant was originally entirely vegan, its menu based on the diet philosophy of an esoteric Christian book called *The Essene Gospel of Peace*, which preached raw foods. Yet the foodie pioneers were far too ahead of their time, and eventually they started serving eggs and dairy to appeal to a wider clientele. Soon, the Source became popular with the "it" crowd of Hollywood, with bohemian celebrity patrons including Joni Mitchell, Warren Beatty, and even John Lennon and Yoko Ono, who ordered the popular "Hi-Protein Salad." But the Source was serving up more than food—as the big sign outside proclaimed, it was cooking up its own New Age philosophy.

The founder, Jim Baker, had a checkered history. Born in Ohio in 1922, he ended up in Los Angeles after the Second World War in search of work as a bodybuilder and stuntman. As a teenager, he had befriended Paul Bragg, of Bragg's Apple Cider Vinegar, another charismatic character with a tendency to exaggerate. When Baker got to La La Land, Bragg introduced him to fasting, juicing, intense exercise, and vegetarianism. As the food writer Jonathan Kauffman explains in his book *Hippie Food*: "Hippie food was a rejection . . . as much as it was an embrace of new ingredients and new flavors. Eating brown rice was a political act, just as wearing your hair long or refusing to shave your armpits could subject you to ridicule and harassment."

Baker had an infamously short fuse. In 1955, he accidentally killed his neighbor in Topanga Canyon after an argument involving the neighbor's dog. Managing to avoid prosecution on the grounds of self-defense, Baker and his wife, Elaine, opened two restaurants—the Aware Inn and the Old World, endeavoring to bring vegetarian fare to the masses. But before long, Baker's temper got the better of him again, and he killed another man during a confrontation over the man's young wife.

Jim and Elaine's marriage did not survive the trial, and he hooked up with Dora, a young bohemian Frenchwoman. The two began boozing and taking psychedelics, going without sleep for days, and stealing money from the Old World, the restaurant Baker kept after his divorce. At some point, Baker hit rock bottom and had a spiritual awakening. He decided to open a restaurant influenced by his newfound spiritual passion. Dora soon left him, but Baker met a nineteen-year-old named Robin whom he married despite being decades older.

The Source epitomized the now classic stereotype of the cultish meat-free restaurant. Servers wore long, flowing garments and took kundalini classes with the newly arrived Sikh guru Yogi Bhajan (the one you may have seen on Yogi Tea packages). Rumor has it that when Baker attended his first class with the master, he tried the famous Breath of Fire, a rapid pulsating breathwork, and experienced an altered state of consciousness in which he discovered his inner guru, and soon adopted the moniker "Father Yod." The Source Restaurant became "the Source Family," which by all accounts was a cult. Most of its members were young people searching for spiritual salvation, or perhaps simply for a father figure amid the intergenerational tensions of the era.

The restaurant gradually morphed into a profitable front for the cult. All the members worked long hours but did not earn individual wages. Their earnings and possessions were redirected back into the "family." Father Yod bought a white Rolls-Royce and paraded around town looking like a cross between a Hindu priest and a renegade cowboy. Everywhere he went he was surrounded by young women dressed like forest nymphs, with long hair and flowing robes, some of them pregnant with the many children born into the polyamorous cult during its heyday. The young men looked like hippie versions of the *Lord of the Rings* elves.

Just three years after the restaurant opened, Father Yod decided that all the family members should live together. They found a twenty-four-bedroom mansion in Los Feliz and the tribe of more than a hundred white-clad members with ethereal names like Mercury, Venus, Lotus,

Infinity, Magus, and Electra—all with the last name Aquarian, which they legally changed—moved in. They spent their days doing morning meditations, smoking marijuana (called the "sacred herb"), playing rock-and-roll music, practicing free love, staring at the sun, and of course, following a strictly vegan diet. Many were raw vegans, and even the restaurant's food was not considered "pure" enough. They cut fresh fruit every morning but never let it sit too long for fear of its becoming "devitalized."

Before long, Father Yod faced his downfall. Predictably, it started when he decided to break his marital vow to Robin and take thirteen "spiritual wives" (called the Council of Women), teaching them "Sex Magic." But the partying, drug use, and their psychedelic rock-and-roll band YaHoWha got so out of control that they were kicked out of the mansion for disturbing neighbors. After that, they were pursued by law enforcement due to the presence of underage women, leading the most loyal followers to escape with Father Yod to Hawaii. By the time Woody Allen parodied the restaurant, Father Yod had already died in a hang-gliding accident in Oahu, a day the Source Family calls Black Monday.

After their leader's passing, the "family" dispersed, but the legacy of the cult, and especially its food, lingers in popular culture. As the *Los Angeles Times* quipped at the time, "Whether you see Father Yod as a spiritual visionary who was ahead of his time or a con artist appropriating another culture's traditions so he could sleep with much younger women, the Source Family—and its restaurant—left its mark on Southern California."

———

Fast-forward fifty years, and across town from where the Source restaurant stood in Hollywood is Abbot Kinney Boulevard, which epitomizes the Venice, California, vibe: a unique blend of laid-back skateboard and surf culture, bohemian counterculturalism, and an undeniable sheen of glamour. As I rode on my beach bike along the boulevard's wide expanse, I passed yoga studios, cafés offering matcha and mushroom brews, and high-end shops selling organic cotton clothing, rose gold jewelry, and crystals.

I was on my way to meet one of the pioneering chefs of modern vegan cuisine, a New York transplant named Matthew Kenney, chef of his flagship restaurant, Plant Food & Wine. The restaurant stands at the far end of the street, closest to the beach. No large sign declares the dawn of the Age of Aquarius here. In fact, its sign is easily missed, as its exterior is minimalist. The interior design cannot be more of a contrast with the Source. Instead of the dowdy earth tones of yesteryear, we find monochromatic gray walls, marble tabletops, and a backyard patio set in a serene Zen-like garden. When the sun sets, the fairy lights adorning the communal table give the setting a sense of bohemian chicness.

As I sat down to wait for Kenney, I browsed the menu. No hummus or sprouts in sight. Instead, here you're promised cauliflower bisque with porcini mushrooms and hazelnuts. Beet tartare with pickled radish, herbs, and asparagus. Kimchi dumplings with sesame, ginger, and coriander. Smashed avocado on za'atar flatbread with capers and lemon. Sea bean Caesar salad with nori. Cacio e pepe with kelp noodles, black pepper olives, and pea leaves. Chickpea frittata with market greens and shaved roots. Oyster mushroom with yuzu kosho, cabbage, furikake, and barley. And for dessert? Coconut and banana cream pie.

In true Venice fashion, Kenney arrived on his skateboard. With his youthful energy, sun-kissed olive complexion, and passion for being on the move (he takes calls while riding his bike around the neighborhood), Kenney hardly seems like a chef at all. His vibe is perfectly suited to the West Coast, yet his charm belies an inner East Coast intensity. Kenney was born in a quaint seaside town off the coast of Maine. There wasn't much to do, so Kenney learned to entertain himself through his vivid imagination. Even as he got older, he'd jump on his motorcycle, go to a quiet place, and just daydream.

Food at home was typical Maine fare—seafood, fresh seasonal produce, and local maple syrup. Kenney wanted all the same foods as other American kids—muffins, macaroni and cheese, pizza. He became conscious about nutrition only when he began playing sports and found that cutting out dairy made him feel better. But he never imagined subsisting solely on plant foods. One summer after college at the University of Maine, Kenney took a job at a harbor restaurant, thinking maybe he'd apply to law school. When he didn't get in, he thought about moving to New York.

But that summer, he happened to fall in love with a co-worker at the restaurant. They decided to escape to Hawaii for a few months with only enough money to rent a little cottage with no electricity. They worked odd jobs—he on a banana farm and his girlfriend at a café. They'd go running down to the beach every night and dreamed of their futures in the Big Apple. Kenney found his mind wandering to the city's glamorous restaurant scene. The lovers arrived in the city in the middle of January, freezing after their island paradise, and found a tiny studio on Sixty-seventh Street, between Second and Third avenues.

Kenney's first job was at Christie's, the auction house. One day on his lunch break, he was walking through the neighborhood and stumbled upon an Italian restaurant. "It was really beautiful and small; the menu was fascinating, and it was like poetry to me." He walked in and told the owner he wanted to open a restaurant. The old Italian man seemed skeptical, but he said, "Then you'd better learn to cook," and promptly offered him a job in the kitchen. The experience was a "trial by fire." "I hadn't even been taught how to use a knife properly, and here I was at this grill of this hot New York restaurant, and you know what? I loved it. It was incredible." He found the experience exhilarating and knew he'd stumbled on his version of right livelihood.

Eventually, the pastry chef suggested he get formal training at the French Culinary Institute (now the International Culinary Center). He signed up, without leaving the job. He'd go to culinary school at seven in the morning, and in the evenings, he'd be back at the Italian restaurant six nights a week. "I had no life, but it was worth it," Kenney recalls. He loved everything about the chef life, except for the unhealthiness of the food. All the techniques he learned in culinary school relied heavily on butter and cream. On his breaks, he'd see other culinary students outside smoking and drinking Diet Cokes, and it bothered him. "Chefs should be producers of health, not of illness. I saw the grotesque portions of food they served, and it made me so sad."

A few years later, Kenney got the chance to open his own restaurant, and he knew exactly what he wanted to do: bring together his love of healthful Mediterranean food with the French techniques he'd learned in culinary school. Matthew's was born, and it thrived. His partner got a job in editing, and the pair decided to settle down and get married. Kenney continued to labor at the restaurant and develop his technique. But about nine years in, tragedy struck: an electrical fire caused so much damage to the restaurant that it was too costly to fix. The fire happened around 9/11, after which the whole restaurant scene took a hit in the city. And as if that wasn't enough, Kenney and his wife began to grow apart, separated by their grueling work schedules.

Overwhelmed with stress, Kenney turned to yoga, sometimes practicing twice a day. As he got more into the health scene, a friend introduced him to a raw vegan restaurant in New York City. He took his new girlfriend at the time, a graduate of the same culinary school named Sarma Melngailis. "It was a weird little place. No music, no wine, not much décor. But it was a rainy Monday night, and the place was full. And it was these super-healthy-looking people. Honestly, I found the food didn't taste that good, but the concept was intriguing. I thought, if somebody can make it good and make it cool, this could be the hottest new concept."

Kenney left that restaurant that night high on life and decided to go raw vegan overnight. "My friends probably thought I was crazy, but when I was introduced to raw food, I totally seized on the concept. I thought, this is exactly what the food of the future could be if someone took this philosophy and applied classic techniques of gourmet cooking to plants." Originally, he had wanted to open a French Moroccan restaurant, but now, convinced that cooking food took away some of its vital nutrients, he persuaded his investor to fund this new "raw" approach instead. It turned out there was a big appetite for what would soon be known as "clean eating" in early 2000s New York City, and he and Melngailis decided to collaborate on a new venture: Pure Food & Wine.

Despite struggling through the winter (it turns out nobody wants to eat raw when it's snowing outside), the restaurant prevailed, attracting celebrity clients (Alec Baldwin met his wife at the restaurant) and media buzz. Kenney and Melngailis got a cookbook deal and became the new "it" couple in the New York health food scene. "All of a sudden it was kind of my launch into the plant-based world." Newspapers began running stories about the couple, the two embodying the new glamorized vegan image: svelte figures, lustrous hair, glowing skin.

Yet behind the glitz and the glamor, there was a darker reality. By the time Kenney and Melngailis had their book party, their tensions had escalated to a breakup. Kenney had already decided to part ways from Melngailis and open his own restaurant. Melngailis kept Pure Food & Wine, but bizarrely, she tarnished the restaurant's reputation (and her own) when she and her new boyfriend embezzled money from the restaurant and ended up in prison (Melngailis is the subject of the Neflix documentary *Bad Vegan*). Kenney doesn't like commenting on that experience, but it was a difficult lesson in mixing the personal and professional.

Kenney moved on to making his vision a reality—a global company that would expand into education, products, and licensing. It was clear, too, that he wanted to make his way to California, where people were more open to the plant-based concept. Eventually, he opened Plant Food & Wine, a variation on the name of the previous restaurant. Within a few years, he not only got the restaurant up and running but crafted an entire culinary empire, including a brick-and-mortar cooking school called Plant Lab, multiple cookbooks, and a licensing program to create partnerships with other restaurant founders.

No doubt, Kenney has made mistakes over the years. He feels he probably should have gotten an MBA, because being an innovative chef and a successful businessman are two different things. Claims of unpaid rent and unpaid staff have followed him around the world. Kenney admits himself that his expansion strategy has been aggressive and sometimes he's done things too rashly. In his memoir, he describes himself as a "deal junkie," with his grand ideas sometimes colliding, painfully, with reality. But there is no doubt that like many visionaries, Kenney is trying to do something ambitious: "crafting the future of food."

———————

Kenney is not the first chef to put vegetables at the center of the plate. At the turn of the millennium in 2001, the celebrated French chef Alain Passard provoked backlash from the culinary establishment when he took meat and fish off the menu at L'Arpège, his Michelin-three-starred restaurant in Paris.[1] Describing the end of his love affair with meat in his characteristically poetic way, he commented: "I dedicated nearly thirty years of my life to meat-based cuisine, but I read the last page of that marvelous book."[2]

Back in 2001, the decision was truly revolutionary, especially in France, the birthplace of gastronomy. And as everyone knows, animal products are central to French cuisine, not only in whole cuts of animal flesh, but in everything from sauces and reductions to classic pastries. Those who frequented L'Arpège at the time of Passard's radical decision thought he had gone completely mad. "People would come, sit down, and look at the menu and say, What is this food? And some left."[3] At the time, nutritional guidelines still considered vegetarianism harmful to health. As late as 2015, the French Ministry of Health stated on their website:

> If you eliminate all animal products from your diet, not only all meat products but also eggs and dairy products, be aware that this type of diet makes it difficult to satisfy your needs for essential amino acids, iron, calcium, and certain vitamins. Following a plant-based diet [régime végétalien] over the long term poses health risks, especially for children.[4]

Even though food production is heavily industrialized in France, many French people still imagine that their food comes from old-world farmers in green fields, tending to their animals.[5] Removing animal products is perceived as a loss of culture, with food being an important part of French identity. While living in France, I remember once catching a program on television called "Should We Stop Eating Meat?"[6] Drawing on French nostalgia, one of the guests implored, "Imagine the world we would be in—a world without meat, without cheese, there are no farms, there are no traditions. We will need to throw out thousands of years of culture. French gastronomy will disappear." To this, perhaps the best-known French vegan journalist, Ayméric Caron, responded that cultural traditions are not sacred, and that if they are immoral, they should evolve.

While Passard was challenging one of the central pillars of French culture, his emphasis on growing ingredients locally made him one of the pioneers of the "farm-to-table" concept, which has long been a central part of gastronomy. Much of the restaurant's produce comes from Bois Giroult, a 3.6-hectare garden outside a château in the countryside west of Paris, in the Normandy region. Along with two other farms, these gardens supply the entirety of the fruits and vegetables around which the L'Arpège seasonal menu is based. The gardens are not only entirely organic but use no pesticides or machinery. Passard eventually decided to put some fish and chicken back on the menu, but it remains centered on vegetables. He commented, "We can go back to using produce where behind each product there is an artisan, good farmers, and we will return to a much more sober type of cuisine. For L'Arpège, we will continue our mission, which is to respect nature and respect the seasons, to respect the magnificent poetry that nature has written." *Touché.*

Since then, things have begun changing rapidly in the gastronomic capital of the world. When I visited a few years ago, I was surprised to learn that the world-class Shangri-La Hotel was offering an entirely vegan high tea, which included buttery scones, whipped cream, and all sorts of high-end pastries. The pastry chef, Michael Bartocetti, had previously worked with the world-renowned Michelin-starred chef Alain Ducasse, who is known for having drastically reduced meat on his menus as well. Bartocetti saw the creation of pastries free of animal products as a creative challenge. As he told me when I came to the hotel to interview him: "We wanted to make something that is vegan, but also for those who are not vegan to enjoy the gourmet life, the colors, the aesthetics, and I had to start from scratch. The most difficult part was the replacement of the eggs." While Bartocetti is not himself vegan, and he didn't think France would ever become a vegan nation—"Go to Normandy and tell them to stop eating butter, there will be a civil war"—he represents a new era in French cuisine.

It took a while for the *Guide Michelin* to catch up, but in 2021, it awarded its first Michelin star to an entirely vegan restaurant, and to the shock of many, it was in France. The chef, Claire Vallée, had opened ONA five years before near Bordeaux. Forgoing the French gourmet classics like boeuf bourguignon (beef stew), coq au vin (braised chicken), and blanquette de veau (veal ragout), ONA serves dishes with ingredients like fir, sake, dulse seaweed, and lemongrass. Vallée is among an emerging generation of French chefs who are daring to question the status quo of gourmet cuisine, many inspired by environmentalism and animal ethics, which has a small yet passionate presence in France.

The pandemic was undoubtedly challenging for the restaurant industry globally, but it also provided an opportunity for some to try something new. In 2020, Eleven Madison Park in New York City announced that it would reopen with an entirely plant-based menu. For a restaurant known for dishes such as suckling pig, sea urchin, and lavender-glazed duck, that was big news, and yet all their seats were sold out instantly.[7] The head chef, Daniel Humm, commented to the *New York Times*: "Our idea of what luxury is had to change. We couldn't go back to doing what we did before."[8]

Each of these pioneering chefs has their own philosophy of how to innovate with vegetables. Some, like Passard and Kenney, believe in showcasing fruits and vegetables in their natural glory rather than preparing them to resemble animal-based foods. To Kenney, using soy or seitan, or even processing peas or mung beans to create meat analogues, simply misses the point of culinary innovation. As Kenney said, "My motivation is to develop the techniques that best work for plants. A lot of people talk about vegan food as being boring, but it's exactly the opposite. It's incredibly vibrant. It's all about presentation and technique and flavor, and it could be very cutting edge."

Over on the other side of Los Angeles, the vegan chef Tal Ronnen has a different philosophy about how to make plant-based cuisine appealing. Formerly a personal chef to Oprah Winfrey and Ellen DeGeneres, the Israeli-born chef now runs Crossroads Kitchen, whose contrast to Plant Food & Wine is obvious not only in the food but also the décor. The interior is dimly lit and features dark wood paneling, a long bar, and plush red-cushioned seating in circular booths, evoking an old-time Hollywood nightclub. In contrast to Kenney, Ronnen uses plants to replicate the flavors and textures of traditional foods, thereby rendering animal products irrelevant. As he told me a few years ago, "We want to create foods that people do not think are possible."

Ronnen's spaghetti carbonara, for example, features a "vegan egg yolk" made of whipped yellow tomato béarnaise sauce, which pours out onto the pasta when punctured with a fork. Their "carrot lox" is made by smoking heirloom carrots over hickory, caking them in nori to give them a seafood flavor and then shaving them thinly onto a bagel topped with almond-based cream cheese (Ronnen is cofounder of Kite Hill and Impossible Foods). Or take the "seafood tower" Ronnen created with chef Scot Jones: instead of lobster, they used lobster mushrooms; in place of calamari they used hearts of palm; and for oysters, they used shiitake mushrooms poached in olive oil and cradled in artichoke leaves.

Yet no matter their divergent philosophies, all these chefs reflect an attempt to shift the food paradigm from the traditional model of French culinary cuisine, known for its thick butter-based sauces and meat-heavy dishes, to a more cosmopolitan and creative cuisine. As Kenney said at the end of our many interviews, "We need the right chefs to innovate at the cutting edge of flavor. I think the food paradigm is going to shift—plants will become the center of the plate. I am not predicting a completely vegan society, but I believe all restaurants will be moving to dishes that showcase vegetables." For too long, vegetables have played second fiddle. The time has come for them to take center stage.

———

On the day we met, Kenney generously offered me lunch. Without even looking at the menu, I knew exactly what I wanted to try: his iconic Raw Zucchini Lasagna with Heirloom Tomatoes. The dish is a holdover from the New York restaurant, when Kenney was still making entirely raw food. Instead of traditional pasta sheets, zucchini slices cut razor thin are layered between seasoned heirloom tomatoes and pillowy macadamia nut ricotta made in-house and adorned with a silky green sauce. When the dish arrived, I took a minute to take in the pleasing presentation. Then I took a slow, intentional bite. The zucchini was delicate and fresh, the heirloom tomatoes deeply flavorful, and the macadamia ricotta satisfyingly creamy. I marveled at the culinary skill, but also the contrast between Kenney's craft and the Beyond Burger, which I tried only a few weeks before. Whereas the burger had a for-the-masses mainstream appeal, the zucchini lasagna embodied a kind of aspirational aesthetic, a promise of what plants could be if they were elevated to the heights of gourmet cuisine.

The next time I passed through Los Angeles, I asked Kenney if I could come by to see the dish made from scratch. Kenney graciously agreed and connected me with his head chef, Andre Oliviera. Oliviera had gotten his start in the Kenney empire only three years before, at the bar. He quickly moved to the kitchen and worked his way up to head chef. When I arrived, as agreed, at three thirty, dinner service was set to begin in just half an hour and the kitchen was bustling with all the cooks rushing to be ready in time. Everything is made daily, since raw or lightly cooked food doesn't keep for long.

Oliviera set up his workstation, which featured a large green zucchini, a red heirloom tomato, a pesto made with local California pistachios, a fresh tomato sauce, and the signature macadamia nut ricotta. Oliviera brought over a mandolin—a tool that cuts vegetables razor thin—and set to work. He cut the zucchini in half, trimmed the sides, and then proceeded to slice it into a dozen squares. He placed a pristine white plate down in front of him and embellished it with a green olive oil sauce, the first brush strokes on a blank canvas.

Next, Oliviera carefully arranged the trio of sauces in a triangle right in the center, serving each from a plastic piping bag, and placed three thin zucchini slices on top, followed by a thick slice of tomato. He repeated the process another couple of times, carefully stacking each layer and shaping a beautiful tower of green, white, and red, reminiscent of an Italian flag. The whole process took only a few minutes. I asked Oliviera whether he ever gets tired of making the lasagna, as it's always on the menu. "Surprisingly I don't; it's one of the fun things to make. This is one of the first dishes I learned in the kitchen, and I still have fun with it."

As he labored, Oliviera was gracious enough to answer my many questions. I asked him where the zucchinis and tomatoes were sourced. He explained that the restaurant partners with as many local farms as possible, and they often shop at the Santa Monica Farmers Market. The only ingredient that isn't local, he explained, is the macadamia nuts. The nut originally hails from Australia, but most of its commercial production is now concentrated in Hawaii, since the trees prefer subtropical climates. There, orchards are planted with grafted seedlings but are susceptible to pests and shifting weather patterns due to climate change, which is why macadamias are so expensive. I imagine Kenney gravitated to the nut for its rich, cushiony density, which makes it an ideal substitute for ricotta cheese.

Oliviera had never even heard of plant-based cooking before he started working at Plant Food & Wine, but as he learned the repertoire, it changed his views on food. "You must rethink what good food can be. I worked in many other kitchens before, and regardless of where you go, it's all the same, the same meat-based dishes at every place. But here, it was a tougher challenge, but also more fun. You have to think outside the box and think of dishes that cater not only to the vegans but to everyone. I'm convinced now that this is the future of food."

Chefs play a critical role in elevating veganism onto a cultural pedestal, which has been essential to its growing appeal. But for many, high-end vegan food such as I have described in this chapter can seem out of touch, even exclusionary. The history of veganism is not only about the quest for the cultural limelight, but also a radical struggle against oppression. I wanted to learn more about that part of the movement's history—one that is too often ignored.

Chapter Ten

Soul Food

I think there's a connection between the way we treat animals
and the way we treat people at the bottom of the hierarchy.

—Angela Davis

In the 1960s, an aspiring comedian named Richard "Dick" Gregory
protested alongside Dr. Martin Luther King Jr., Malcolm X, Stokeley
Carmichael, and H. Rap Brown in the civil rights movement. During one
march in Mississippi, a sheriff kicked his wife, who was pregnant at the
time, and he didn't come to her defense. "I was telling myself," says Gregory,
"that the only reason that I didn't fight back was because I was nonviolent.
And then I decided that if I'm nonviolent, and I won't hurt a person, then
animals should get the same respect. At that point, I didn't know nothing
about vegetarianism. I never heard of the word." Yet in 1965, he became
one.[1] "Animals and humans suffer and die alike. Violence causes the same
pain, the same spilling of blood, the same stench of death, the same arro-
gant, cruel, and brutal taking of life."

A few of years later, Gregory ran for the mayor of Chicago. During his
campaign, a supporter named Dr. Alvenia M. Fulton came by headquarters to drop off nutritious salads for him and his staff. Although he didn't

end up winning the race, Gregory tracked her down to express his thanks. He discovered that Dr. Fulton was a naturopath, passionate about fasting and following a plant-based diet for health and wellness. In the 1950s, she ran the Better Living Health Club from her home, and she eventually opened Fultonia's Health Food Center on Chicago's south side, a restaurant that served soups, vegetarian chilis, brown rice, salads, fruit platters, vegetable juices, whole grain breads, and wholesome cakes. The connection turned out to be the beginning of a fruitful collaboration.

Dr. Fulton introduced Gregory to fasting, something he had been wanting to try, given his knowledge of Gandhi's fasts for social justice. Gregory was looking to "do something dramatic and personal to protest the continued slaughter in Vietnam," and a long fast, at least one month, seemed like just the right kind of thing. And so, from Thanksgiving of 1967 through to New Year's Day of 1968, Gregory went on his first forty-day fast with the assistance of Dr. Fulton. By the end, Gregory's weight had dropped from 280 pounds to a mere 97, while he maintained his grueling comedy show schedule. He quipped, "I've lost so much weight that nonviolence is no longer a tactic, it's a necessity."

Gregory didn't lose any time promoting his way of life. For a while, he was giving almost 250 lectures a year on college campuses across the country, inspiring many young Black Americans. In his 1973 book *Dick Gregory's Natural Diet for Folks Who Eat: Cookin' with Mother Nature*, his comedic nature shines through in chapter titles such as "Warning: The Author Has Determined That Not Reading the Following Pages Is Dangerous to Your Health." But the light tone belies a serious message. He writes that what we eat is at the core of who we are. By giving up animal products and processed foods and embracing instead the gifts offered by Mother Nature, people gain benefits of great value—health, youthful energy, better appearance, and greater mental clarity.

Yet for Gregory, as for many others, the biggest rewards aren't material, but spiritual. He describes his slow progression from a vegetarian diet to a vegan one, and eventually to a fruitarian diet consisting of fresh fruits and vegetables, with the help of Dr. Fulton. "What began as an act of social protest—a political act—became in the process of living it a 'purifying act'—in mind, body, and spirit. As my body was cleansed of years of accumulated impurities, my mind and spiritual awareness were lifted to a new level. I felt closer to Mother Nature and all her children. I felt more in tune with the universal order of existence. I was now aware of the words I used to hear in church: *The body is a temple of the spirit.* Just as Jesus drove the moneychangers out of the temple, fasting had driven the devils of my former diet from my own temple and my life changed completely."

———

When I first decided to embrace a vegan lifestyle, I had no idea that the largest vegan demographic (proportionally to the population) in the United States isn't, as many people assume, white and wealthy people living on the coasts, but instead Black Americans. A 2019 Gallup poll found that nearly a third of people of color in America reported cutting down on meat in the previous year, compared to only about one-fifth of white Americans, and more African Americans than white Americans say they follow a strict vegan diet.[2]

How come, I wondered, was this fact is not more widely known? That's the same question that filmmaker Jasmine Leyva wondered about too. When Leyva first became vegan, she felt out of place in a movement that to her, as a young Black American, felt exclusive. Looking around, she wondered, "Why aren't there any black vegans?" The question led her on a journey to make a documentary film called *The Invisible Vegan*, a title inspired by Ralph Ellison's 1952 novel *The Invisible Man*, which explores many of the challenges faced by African Americans in the twentieth century. Like Ellison, who felt invisible not only in white spaces, where he wasn't seen as equal, but also in Black spaces, where he didn't fit certain stereotypes, Leyva says, "That's exactly how I felt as a black vegan."

Growing up in Detroit, she had no knowledge of a plant-based lifestyle until she moved to Los Angeles to pursue a career in filmmaking. One day, she found herself at a vegan restaurant called Stuff I Eat, founded by an astonishingly fit and youthful chef in her seventies named Babette Davis, who's been vegan for thirty years and attributes her appearance and athleticism to her dietary regimen. Inspired, Leyva began reading about the plant-based lifestyle and adopted it immediately.

But when Leyva went home to visit, her friends and family pushed back. "I went home and told my friends about this diet, and they racialized my choice, saying 'Oh so now you're on this Hollywood diet, you're eating all this white people food.' But I was confused because I was inspired by an African American woman." Still, when she considered how rarely Black veganism is represented in the mainstream media, it clicked. Not only did Leyva feel she didn't fit the image of a "vegan" as popular culture represented it, but she also didn't see the hard work of activists of color being acknowledged.

The writer and entrepreneur Amirah Mercer had a similar experience renouncing pork, which she used to see as a "life-giving food," in favor of a plant-based diet. In a beautifully poetic piece called "A Homecoming" for *Eater*, she explains how the imagery of whiteness and thinness promoted by the wellness industry led her to believe that veganism wasn't for her. "The way we cooked and ate—sharing freely with anyone who stopped by—felt unique to Black culture, and my veganism initially seemed like a rebuke of the rituals I had known. I felt like I was revoking my own Black card."

The exclusivity of the vegan movement isn't a new phenomenon. As Jonathan Kauffman writes in his book *Hippie Food*:

> The health food movement of the 1970s was stunted by the same problems that hobble the sustainable-food movement fifty years on: longhair circles were almost exclusively white, which left people of color with the burden of adapting to the majority's terms, beliefs, and unconscious prejudices to join. Plus, the food movement was characterized by pervasive nostalgia—a preindustrial romanticism—that was disconcerting and painful to anyone whose ancestors, in that preindustrial era, were slaves.[3]

But the more Mercer learned about veganism in the Black community, the more she realized that her embrace of plants was in fact picking up a long-lost cultural thread. As she puts it, "The imagery of veganism propagated by the wellness industry erases the long—and often radical—history of plant-based diets in the Black diaspora."[4] Mercer learned that several prominent civil rights leaders besides Dick Gregory, including Rosa Parks, Coretta Scott King, and her son with Dr. King, Dexter Scott King, embraced vegetarianism and veganism, not to mention many other Black politicians and intellectuals including Alice Walker, Pulitzer Prize–winning author of *The Color Purple*, and the scholar and activist Angela Davis. Today, the politicians Senator Cory Booker and New York City mayor Eric Adams are vocal about their own motivations for veganism.

Explaining her views on veganism at the 27th Empowering Women of Color Conference held at UC Berkeley in 2012, Davis commented: "I usually don't mention that I'm vegan, but that has evolved. I think it's the right moment to talk about it because it is part of a revolutionary perspective—how can we not only discover more compassionate relations with human beings but how can we develop compassionate relations with the other creatures with whom we share this planet and that would mean challenging the whole capitalist industrial form of food production."[5] She went on: "The food we eat masks so much cruelty. The fact that we can sit down and eat a piece of chicken without thinking about the horrendous conditions under which chickens are industrially bred in this country is a sign of the dangers of capitalism, how capitalism has colonized our minds."

Today, many icons of Black culture follow a plant-based lifestyle: Stevie Wonder, Questlove, stic.man of the rap duo Dead Prez, Cardi B, Lizzo, and most of the members of the group Wu-Tang Clan, as well as tennis star sisters Serena and Venus Williams. Even Beyoncé and Jay-Z began to offer a plant-based meal planning service a few years ago in partnership with their former personal trainer Marco Borges. When I interviewed Borges at the Waldorf Astoria in Beverly Hills, he explained that after adopting a plant-based diet while training the pair, he suggested they try it too. "I said he would do it for his birthday through Christmas and B said, I'll do it too." At the precise moment Borges and I met for our interview, Beyoncé just happened to drop a picture of a vegan avocado toast breakfast muffin on her Instagram feed, offering concert tickets to fans who pledged to adopt a plant-based diet. Borges's phone exploded with texts, and we had to postpone the interview for the next day.

These musicians and athletes are motivated by a myriad of reasons, but one of the most common is health. As the pandemic painfully showed, there are huge health disparities between African Americans and their white counterparts. Many Black Americans suffer from chronic conditions such as obesity, hypertension, gout, diabetes, and other ailments that can be traced back to the Western (and many would say colonial) diet, and this reality was keenly felt during the COVID-19 pandemic.[6] Medical scares have led many to realize their mortality and take their health more seriously. But for others, embracing a plant-based diet meant renouncing a familiar way of eating that for them represents home: "soul food."

———

"Soul food" has a complex history. In his book *Hog and Hominy: Soul Food from Africa to America*, the food historian Frederick Douglass Opie explains that "soul food originated in the quarters of enslaved Africans in the sixteenth to nineteenth centuries. It is a blend, or a creolization, of many cooking traditions that Africans across the Americas seasoned to their own definition of perfection with their knowledge of culinary herbs gained from their ancestors." Opie writes that the term itself dates to the 1920s, with the "chitlin circuit"—the string of black-owned honky-tonks, nightclubs, and theaters.

But it was only in the 1960s, at the height of the civil rights movement, that "soul food" became its own cuisine. In a 1966 essay, Amiri Baraka (formerly LeRoi Jones) put forth the idea of "soul food" as an African American cultural invention, declaring "hog maws, chitlins, sweet potato pie, pork sausage and gravy, fried chicken or chicken in the basket, barbecued ribs, hopping John, hush puppies, fried fish, hoe cakes, biscuits, salt pork, dumplings, and gumbo all came directly out of the black belt region of the South and represented the best of African American cookery."[7]

These sentiments gave people a sense of pride around their food and inspired them to write soul food cookbooks and open soul food restaurants. Predictably, this group of home cooks and chefs eventually faced a backlash from white intellectuals who believed soul food was part of a broader Southern regional culture. Other criticism came from Black Americans whom Opie calls "food rebels," who insisted that soul food was nothing to celebrate since it was leading to sickness and death in the Black community.

Dick Gregory was among the critics. Disparaging soul food in his book, he wrote, "I personally would say that the quickest way to wipe out a group of people is to put them on a soul food diet. One of the tragedies is that the very folks in the black community who are most sophisticated in terms of the political realities in this country are nonetheless advocates of 'soul food.' They will lay down a heavy rap on genocide in America with regard to black folks, then walk into a soul food restaurant and help the genocide along."

These health rebels were continuing the legacy of pioneers like George Washington Carver, a legendary African American who was born into slavery but rose to become an agricultural scientist, inventor, and environmentalist. Carver taught at the Tuskegee Institute and became famous for his role in promoting peanuts as a widely available, cheap protein, out of which he created early iterations of products that imitated chicken, duck, and nondairy milk. Far before his time, Carver believed that plant foods held the secret to health and longevity for the Black community.

Many of these critics argued that "soul food" was born not of cultural expression but of oppression. African Americans did what they could do with the food they had available, which, on plantations, often meant cornmeal and the parts of pigs considered least desirable, such as chitterlings (intestines), hog maws, and pig's feet. Bringing culinary creativity to bear, many enslaved people managed to turn these foodstuffs into mainstays and even delicacies of Southern cooking today. But in the longer arc of African

American history, soul food has its origins in the staples eaten in West Africa for generations.

In *High on the Hog*, a book that became a Netflix special, the food historian Jessica B. Harris explains that many of the vegetables and fruits often associated with African Americans—sweet potatoes, black-eyed peas, okra, watermelon—are those that survived the transatlantic journey.[8] Okra, for example, is prized in Nigerian cuisine for its thickening properties, while watermelon originated in ancient Egypt. Black-eyed peas, which are a key component of hopping John, the dish that is supposed to bring good luck on New Year's Day, were cultivated in Central Africa and are considered lucky in many West African cultures. Sweet potatoes (called "yams" in the South, a holdover from a long-ago era) and cassava are indispensable starches in many African cuisines.

The emphasis on "soul food" in the United States misses the broader tapestry of food culture in the African diaspora around the world, and the strikingly consistent thread of natural plant-based diets. As the chef Jenné Claiborne opens in her cookbook *Sweet Potato Soul*, "My great-grandparents from the South—and my ancestors from West Africa—ate a mostly plant-based diet because it is efficient, reliable, and nutritious." Claiborne's father had grown up in an African Hebrew Israelite community, which preaches a vegan diet. In the 1960s, members of the sect began emigrating to Israel with their leader Ben Ammi Ben-Israel (born Ben Carter), believing that they were descendants of the Ten Lost Tribes of Israel.[9] Taking inspiration from the Bible, they adopted a plant-based diet as the secret to regenerative health and spiritual salvation.

When I came to Israel a few years ago to understand the sudden rise of veganism in the tiny country, I learned that many vegan Israelis had first been exposed to the idea of a *tivonoot* (deriving from the Hebrew word *teva*, "nature") diet from the Black community, which runs restaurants across the country serving mushroom and black lentil burgers, whole wheat vegan quiches, and fruit purées. Every Shabbat the African Hebrew Israelite community fasts, and four times a year they spend a whole week eating only raw foods. As Nir Avieli, an anthropologist at Ben-Gurion University who's been studying the community for over a decade, sums up in an interview with *Haaretz*,[10] the African Hebrew Israelites' regimen is "related to their world view about repairing the injustice caused to the enslaved peoples. The body can be a slave, but the soul will remain free. The basic assumption is that Creation is perfect; all that is needed is to be cleansed of man's injustices, whether those caused to the black man in Africa or the injustices of mankind in general."

A similar philosophical and spiritual vein runs through the Ital cuisine of Jamaica, which was created by Rastafarians and is almost entirely plant-based and emphasizes fresh, organic fruits and vegetables and raw food. My personal exposure to this cuisine was abroad, in Paris, where I stumbled into a vegan Ital restaurant called Jah Jah and interviewed its owner, a strikingly beautiful woman with long red curls named Coralie Jouhier. Her mother is from Martinique and her father from Senegal, and she cofounded the restaurant with her partner, Daqui Gomis. Inspired by the foods they grew up with on the island, they serve comforting bowls filled to the brim with spicy black-eyed peas, rice jollof, fried plantains, hot dogs consisting of brioche buns (a nod to the French) filled with beechwood-smoked carrot "sausage," and coconut cream cake for dessert.

In 2011, the nonprofit Oldways, which tries to help people rediscover healthful and sustainable ways of eating across different cultural traditions, included an African Heritage Diet among their food pyramids, modeled like the Standard American Diet food pyramid of the USDA. Although the pyramid includes some animal products, its emphasis is on grains, beans, vegetables, and spices. A section entitled "Change the Way You Think About Meat" includes advice such as "Use lean, healthy meats in smaller amounts for flavor," "Make rice and beans your new staple," and "With the zesty flavors of African heritage, you may not even notice the meat's not there."

———

One of the people leading the renaissance of a new and health-conscious "black food" is the vegan chef Bryant Terry, whom I met in Oakland,

California. Terry believes that "soul food" based on whole plant foods is actually more authentic to the origins of the culinary African diaspora. "For most people," he writes in his cookbook *Vegan Soul Kitchen*, "African American and Southern cooking is synonymous with meals organized around fatty meats with overcooked vegetables and fruits playing a minor supporting role." Think fried chicken, greens, corn bread, rolls, and sweet potato pie. "But," Terry reminds us, "when we take a step back and remember—that before the widespread industrialization of food in this country—African Americans living in the South included lots of fresh, nutrient-dense leafy greens, tubers, and fruits in their everyday diets."[11]

The chef Jenné Claiborne echoes these sentiments: "Black food has historically been vegetarian and has relied most on dark leafy greens (collards, turnip greens, and mustard greens), beans (especially black-eyed peas), whole grains (corn and rice), and starchy vegetables (sweet potatoes, turnips, potatoes). African diets, just like other diets all around the world, have historically been based on starchy root vegetables like yams, greens, and peanuts, and meat was reserved for special occasions. Animal products only became a bigger part of the diet with industrialization and the wider availability of those foods."

For both Terry and Claiborne, the practice of developing vegan soul food recipes isn't just about reconnecting with tradition, bringing health and food education to their people, or culinary creativity, but it's also a broader project to, as Terry writes in *Afro-Vegan*, "move Afro-diasporic food from the margins closer to the center of our collective culinary consciousness and to put its ingredients, cooking techniques, and flavor profiles into wider circulation."

Terry's journey toward health consciousness began in high school when he became a football player and began eating a better diet. But his transition to veganism was inspired by music, which he loves as much as he loves food, specifically an old-school rap song called "Beef" by Boogie Down Productions, which traces the classic American food chain and confronts topics such as antibiotics use, lack of hygiene in slaughterhouses, and chronic disease linked to meat. Like food, Terry believes that music is powerful in shifting people's habits, so in his cookbooks he pairs recipes with suggestions for songs to listen to while cooking, an idea he got from Jessica B. Harris, who suggests musical artists to accompany her menus in her classic cookbook *The Welcome Table: African American Heritage Cooking*. Flipping through Terry's cookbooks, I recognized a few of my own favorite tunes. Growing up with a culturally curious father, I was exposed to all manner of international music, including West African, Cuban, Caribbean, jazz, blues, funk, and reggae. To this day, my ears are often filled with Billie Holiday, Ella Fitzgerald, Louis Armstrong, Miles Davis, Thelonious Monk, Ali Farka Touré, and Toumani Diabaté.

Visiting Terry at his house in Oakland, I smiled when I heard my favorite artist, the Cape Verdean singer Cesaria Evora, singing from the backyard stereo, and somewhere deep in my soul, I felt at home. I saw Evora in concert a couple of times before she died, and she's accompanied my writing ever since high school. For Terry, sharing songs is like sharing good food—both have the power to bring people together. "My goal has always been to cast the widest net and I always go back to that moment when I heard that brilliant song about factory farming and its impacts on animals and the environment and human health, and I remember what an impact it had in shifting my own personal trajectory. It's a powerful lesson in how to educate and move people."

Terry is a central figure putting "black food" into the limelight, but back when he was trying to get his first cookbook published, he got a dozen rejections. "People thought I was cutting the pie too thin. They felt it was an oxymoron to think about veganism and blackness and they just couldn't imagine putting those things together in the same box in their heads." He understood that publishers were crunching numbers on potential sales and felt there couldn't possibly be a market for his concept. But that kind of reaction is exactly why he felt his book needed to exist, to change the dominant cultural narrative and reclaim the ancestral diets of formerly enslaved people. "I think it's important to push back against this narrative because many of my ancestors, and people in the working class, couldn't afford to have meat at every single meal. In that generation, large portions of meat were reserved for holidays and special occasions. In everyday meals, like soups or stews, meat was only used to deepen the flavor."

The song "Beef" mentions a book called *How to Eat to Live*, a two-volume work published in 1967 and 1972 by Elijah Muhammad, founder of the Nation of Islam. For many years, the Black nationalist organization preached a vegetarian diet, among other edicts. Although the Nation of Islam is controversial, its rejection of the "white man's diet" aligned with other African American organizations seeking to bring a healthier lifestyle to their communities, including the Black Panthers' Free Breakfast for School Children program, founded in 1969 by the Black Panther Party in Oakland.

Yet the question of whether—and how—to tell people what to eat is, of course, deeply fraught. Psyche Williams-Forson, a professor of American history and author of *Building Houses out of Chicken Bones*, told me that she often laments wellness approaches to change. "It's this narrative of empowerment, because you know, it's better for people's health. But at the same time, you're taking away people's choices, and it's one of the few things they have control over in their lives . . . So it's a complicated argument because we want to allow people to have the choices to make whether the choice they make is good for them or not." She points out that telling people they have a choice about how to eat implies that, should they choose to eat food deemed unhealthful, they deserve to suffer. She's also concerned about moralizing, and the deep history of white society offering to "help" those they see as not able to help themselves. "My first question is always 'Did you talk to the people in this community? Do they want what you're trying to bring? Do they want to go out of their way to the farmers market when they're being paid minimum wage? Do they want to tend to the garden you're trying to grow?'"

Williams-Forson's complex critique echoes a broader issue within the vegan movement, which concerns exclusivity. In recent years, more critics have pointed out that the dominant narrative of veganism ignores the reality of most people's lives. The vast majority of people cannot afford to drink green juices, eat fresh berries, or buy only organic food. Many don't even have access to such foods. There are also many powerful structural factors at play in determining what people eat, complicating the issue of free choice. While fast food restaurants dot the country, they are especially prominent in poorer areas. A study of more than six thousand fast food restaurants found that they were 60 percent more likely to advertise to children in Black versus white neighborhoods.[12] These advertisements attract kids' attention with cartoon characters, movie stars, sports figures, and 3D cutouts.

These criticisms have a long history in the sociological tradition in which I was trained, stemming back all the way to the work of the French sociologist Pierre Bourdieu, who famously argues that "taste" isn't idiosyncratic, but is shaped by our position in the social hierarchy.[13] That means everything from the music we listen to, the kinds of schools we attend, the jobs we strive for, and the spouses we marry to the art we buy, the home renovation projects we undertake, and even the way we parent signals what lifestyle choices we have access to and which are out of reach. Food "choices" are an especially obvious place where class differences matter. The kind of food we buy, its cultural origins, who prepares it and how, says a lot about our social position. Most "foodies" are from high-status backgrounds, which is why they can afford to treat food as something that is to be enjoyed, even fetishized, rather than as what it is for most people: a necessity.

In the last few years, many foodies have become more concerned with eating food that is not only good-tasting but "good" from an ethical standpoint. One survey of food shoppers in a range of discount and premium grocery stores in Toronto, Canada, showed that while there are ways of consuming ethically (such as being a dumpster-diving "freegan") that are considered low-status, those who combine both aesthetic and ethical considerations into their food choices are considered highest status (measured in terms of education, occupation, and income).[14]

There is undeniable privilege in the vegan movement and many social issues to confront, including the fact that much of the leadership is male, white, and wealthy, even though, as we now know, women[15] and people of color[16] are disproportionately more likely to identify as vegan or plant-based eaters. At the same time, the refrain that veganism is "elitist" is a bizarre twist on history, since it is meat that has long held high status. In the past, meat was hard to get, whereas now factory-farmed meat is omnipresent. In this context, the avoidance of mass-produced meat becomes the new marker of class consciousness.

Paradoxically, though, it's precisely this elitist element that makes veganism aspirational for many. The "vegan glow" derives, in part, from the healthfulness of certain foods, but also from their cultural cachet. In its association with celebrities, athletes, and social media influencers, high-end restaurants, and costly practices such as juice cleanses, veganism has entered a new frontier of cultural representation. Vegans might still be unrelatable, but now that's because they are wealthy, fit, and slim rather than because they are hippies on the fringe. A similar dynamic occurred in the case of yoga, which became popular when it was commodified into a trendy lifestyle complete with branded clothing, high-end studios, and teacher training programs that led to mass adoption.

Today, many leaders of the plant-based movement are not marginal social movement activists but members of the mainstream who found a way to reconfigure the lifestyle to consumer trends. What were once unusual dietary requests are now commonplace, entering the lives of even those who do not practice veganism directly, such as when a relative requests vegan sides at Thanksgiving dinner. Yet the reality is that most of those who promote veganism are privileged on many dimensions. Still, it seems to me that it's possible to promote veganism without necessarily packaging it as a privileged, out-of-reach lifestyle. For many communities, including those in the African American diaspora, plant-based diets offer a chance to rediscover a lost heritage.

As Terry told me, "Many Black people have encountered white vegans who have presented as very dogmatic and judgmental and paternalistic toward Black people. They're not thinking about the cultural aspects of their message, and that's something I see missing from the conversation.

That is why I emphasize ancient culinary traditions and teach people about the cornucopia of delicious and culturally relevant foods that make it possible for people to eat a sustainable and healthy plant-based diet."

Growing up, Terry watched his family members plant dozens of rows of collard greens in the backyard garden he would play in as a child. This "quintessential staple of African American cooking" would be simmered in an enormous steel pot until meltingly soft. Conjuring up a recipe that represents him and his ancestors, he says: "I figured that more than any other food, collards serve as the consummate ambassador for what I imagined as my people's cuisine." Pausing for a moment, he adds, "I want people to realize that collard greens are a superfood!"

That's why Terry is cynical about the "innovations" of Silicon Valley. "I tend to push back against industrialized plant-based meat because I think it's an uncreative and boring approach to eating. I want people to embrace real food and to understand how to prepare real food. The industry wants us to choose convenience and to sacrifice creativity, and a part of me understands that, especially when we have busy lives and kids, but I wonder if we can reimagine the way we think about feeding ourselves, to move past individuality and think about how we can take care of each other and build community by feeding each other." Terry imagines building neighborhood gardens outside churches and schools, where each family contributes something different, such as growing the food, preserving the food, and preparing the food for shared meals. His vision for an ideal food system goes far beyond veganism, to a way of feeding ourselves that weaves back together social fabrics that have been withered away by the industrialized fast-food system.

Such a vision already exists and has a deep history within the African American community. As the culinary historian Michael B. Twitty writes in his book *The Cooking Gene*, "Long before anyone heard of a 'victory garden' [vegetable gardens planted in support of the war effort during World Wars I and II], Africans in America, South and North, were no strangers to the truck patch of provision ground." He explains how many enslaved people kept gardens, growing yams, cassava, rice, millet, sorghum, peppers, greens, and okra. "These spaces were little landscapes of resistance: Resistance against a culture of dehumanizing poverty and want, resistance against the erasure of African cultural practices, resistance against the destruction of African religions, and resistance against slavery itself."[17] As his friend Ron Finley, the "gangsta gardener" of urban Los Angeles, puts it, "Growing food is like growing money."[18]

These conversations reminded me of one I had recently with my downstairs neighbor Jacquie, an African American woman in her sixties whom I've watched tend her garden for a couple of years while living in Oakland. She grows strawberries, figs, lemons, tomatoes, zucchini, kale, and of course collard greens. Occasionally she offers us a sun-kissed cherry tomato to sample, or advice such as boiling mint in hot water to perfume the house. Once she left a baby Sun Gold tomato plant on our porch, which inspired us to start our own balcony garden. On a slow, sunny afternoon in April, I asked her how she learned to garden, and her answer was simple. "Oh, everybody back home"—she's from Georgia—"knows how to garden. I learned just watching my mother, planting seeds, watering, waiting for your food to grow. It's soul food!" Or, as Dr. Fulton put it, "soul food with a mission, and the mission is good health."

What's inspiring about the work of these social reformers is that they are trying not only to start a conversation about veganism and what it means to modern food justice, but also to encourage people from every cultural background to realize that to eat a healthful diet, they need look no further than the food staples of their own culinary history. As Terry says, "All we can do as educators is plant those seeds with the hope that one day that lightbulb moment may happen." And just like Terry, there are those who believe that the key to the future of food lies, paradoxically, in its past.

Chapter Eleven

The Past of Food

Like water that flows through the worlds, serving as it moves along, tofu joyfully surrenders itself to the endless play of transformation. All as if it knew there was no death to die, no fixed or separate self to cling to, no other home than here.

—BILL SHURTLEFF AND AKIKO AOYAGI

A few weeks after I met Bryant Terry, I found myself on the other side of the East Bay, in the sunny kitchen of Minh Tsai. Tsai's house is a classic Berkeley craftsman, at least a hundred years old, with what looked like an original white gas oven, farmhouse sink, and white tiled walls. Tsai is a tofu maker (he often wears a shirt that asks, WHO'S YOUR TOFU MASTER?). On that day, he generously offered to host me for lunch and to show me how to make tofu from scratch.

In his fifties, Tsai exudes boundless energy. He welcomed me into the kitchen cheerily, and I found my place at the island. "Today we're going to make silken tofu!" I'm a pretty good cook, but I was used to buying my tofu premade, usually sealed in plastic, just like everyone else. I knew, of course, that tofu was made of soybeans, but I didn't know what else the process involved. Tsai pulled a large jug of soy milk from the fridge. "I made this earlier, just from ground soybeans. It's the same kind we use at Hodo." Hodo Foods is the company Tsai founded in 2004 after getting his start at local farmers markets. Tsai poured the fresh soy milk into a saucepan and lit the fire. "We're just going to wait for it to get warm."

While we waited, I asked Tsai why he wanted to start a tofu company. "It's kind of cliché because so many people start a food business because they couldn't find something they liked in the marketplace, but that rings true for me." Tsai grew up in Vietnam, to parents of Chinese origin. "I grew up in a society where we buy our food daily, like in Europe. It's very seasonal, and so every day my grandfather and I would get up in the morning and walk down the alleyway and I still remember the smell of soy milk. We would get this hot, sweet milk, and we would also pick up a block of tofu in a plastic bag and bring it home to my grandmother."

Years later, after he had immigrated to the United States, Tsai was working in investment banking when a recession hit. He began thinking about what else he could do. Tsai thought about other kinds of food businesses, maybe wine, but ultimately decided that what he missed most was the good-quality tofu he grew up eating back home. "I remember being disappointed by what I found in stores. The tofu was bland, even at Asian markets. I'd look at the ingredients and wonder, why isn't there quality tofu made with non-GMO soybeans without all these added preservatives?"

It wasn't an easy time to start a tofu business, as the controversy around soy was just beginning to swirl. "When I learned that tofu was one of the most contentious foods in the West, I was so blown away by the misinformation. I mean, I understand soy allergies, but here was this food that's been around for thousands of years with all these health benefits and different flavors and tastes and all of that was being thrown out the window." In the early days, when Tsai was selling his tofu at the market, customers would come up to his stand and tell him that their doctor recommended they eat more soy. They would look at him quizzically, curious to see what he'd say, but Tsai is not the type to convince anyone. "I don't have a tofu agenda. But I was surprised because it's often those people who became my most avid customers."

Yet even as building Hodo Foods was challenging, it paled in comparison to the experience he had at thirteen, when his family was forced to escape Vietnam by boat. Although the Vietnam War never reached Ho Chi Minh City, where they lived, Tsai's family had two strikes against them: after Vietnam chose to align itself with the Soviet Union rather than China during the war, ethnic Vietnamese began to look at Chinese Vietnamese with suspicion, and Tsai and his family were told to leave the country. And as teachers, his parents fell into another mistrusted category: intellectuals. Tsai's parents were ideologically Communists, but they feared for their lives and chose to flee by boat, ultimately landing at a refugee camp in Malaysia. Tsai would later write about the experience in a memoir he amusingly called "Huckleberry Minh," which he wrote for his children.

After six months at the camp, the family heard that an American church would sponsor their move to Maryland. Eventually the family landed in San Francisco, where Tsai's mother became a seamstress and hairdresser and his father delivered newspapers and later became a journalist. Tsai learned English quickly and won scholarships to good schools, including San Francisco University High School in the city's Pacific Heights neighborhood, where he met the children of politicians and corporate leaders. That experience allowed him to see a horizon far beyond his family's enclave. He went on to get both undergraduate and graduate degrees in economics at Columbia University, specializing in developmental economics. By the time he started Hodo Foods, Tsai had already realized the American Dream, but he felt a pull toward entrepreneurship.

In the early 2000s, the Bay Area was experiencing a kind of food renaissance with the farm-to-table movement, and an entire cohort, Tsai among them, launched successful businesses through the vast network of farmers markets. By this time, Tsai had honed his tofu technique, having learned from various masters, and turned the art into a science. After meeting a few investors, Tsai and his small team began to expand and had to figure out how to ship their products to the East Coast. They spent more than two years on the task, learning how to pasteurize tofu to expand its shelf life from twenty to sixty days without changing the ingredients. Tsai stayed true to his commitment to producing the purest tofu he could, without preservatives, like the tofu he ate as a child in Vietnam.

The soy milk was about the right temperature now, and Tsai invited me to join him at the stove. "I'm going to treat you to something which is very rare. This is the freshest yuba you'll ever taste." Yuba, I found out, is the dried skin that forms on top of soy milk, and it's a prized ingredient in Asian cooking. I could see the soy milk frothing, a thin sheet forming over the liquid below. Tsai scooped it up gingerly with a fork and handed it to me. It tasted like a cloud. Suddenly, I was transported to my own childhood in Moldova, into my own grandmother's tiny kitchen, tasting the froth of simmering dairy milk. I remember finding the cow version off-putting, far too sour. But the soy milk has a pleasant frothy sweetness.

Satisfied, Tsai turned off the stove and set a wide aluminum bowl on the kitchen counter. He poured in the soy milk slowly, and then brought over a white powder. "This is a coagulant, which is what binds tofu together. There are three types of coagulants that are currently being used for tofu making, and the most traditional is this one, calcium sulfate, which is basically gypsum, but a diluted form. It's a mineral found in the ground, and this one happens to come from Utah, because that's where it's found in the U.S. The good thing about calcium sulfate is it doesn't mask the flavor of the soybeans, and so that's the one they like in China." Tsai poured the white powder in and then began running a whisk through the mixture, not in the circular motion I was used to from baking, but instead in sharp diagonal strokes. The soy milk began to curdle, absorbing the coagulant.

Tsai explained that when the recipe for tofu reached Japan about a thousand years ago, the Japanese didn't have gypsum, so they had to find another binding agent. They developed nigari, or magnesium chloride, a white powder that is produced when sodium chloride is removed from seawater. The name comes from the Japanese word for "bitter," and Japanese tofu has a slightly bitter flavor compared to the traditional Chinese. These were the only two natural coagulants available for tofu production until the Japanese developed GDL, a synthetic coagulant created through fermentation. Its advantage is that it coagulates much faster and creates a firmer tofu than the traditional variety, allowing it to be packaged, transported, and distributed at scale.

Tsai took out a bamboo box the size of a tofu block and lined it with a soaked cheesecloth. Carefully spooning the tofu chunks into the box, he wrapped it and then handed me the lid of the box. "There, you try." I took the lid and placed it over the tofu, pressing down slowly. "The more you push, the firmer it gets." It took a few minutes, but I managed to drain out most of the excess liquid, and then Tsai refilled the metal bowl with fresh water. "This is the fun part. Take the whole block and put it in the water. It's delicate, and we want it to cool. Then slowly unfold it. Roll up your sleeves, literally," he chuckled.

I transferred the tofu block and peeled back the cheesecloth slowly, until it was almost unwrapped. Tsai swooped in, pulling off the rest with the skilled hand of a magician revealing something hidden beneath a cloth to the audience. The block somersaulted into the water. Bringing over a plate, Tsai gestured for me to again transfer the block. I picked up the warm, soft tofu and carefully placed it on the plate. "It's funny, every time I give a workshop, all the women who've had children say, 'Oh, it's like giving birth.' The warm block reminds them of a newborn."

Tsai told me that in Asia, it's common to see people walking around selling tofu from a bucket. "They'll slice off a thin piece of it for you and put on some savory spices or maybe daikon radish. Or they'll pour some sugary syrup on top as a dessert. It almost tastes like ice cream. Me, I like it with some plain soy sauce." Tsai cut off a thin slice and handed me a bowl of soy sauce. "Try it like that." I put a few drops of soy sauce on top of the jiggly tofu and took a bite. It tasted a little beany, but also surprisingly like a soft cheese, with a sweet aftertaste. "That sweetness is a special part of the tofu, and many people don't get to taste it unless they make it fresh. It really debunks the whole idea that tofu has no flavor. People only think that because they haven't tasted the truly real thing."

The whole process took us only about twenty minutes, with soy milk prepared in advance. Soy milk, it turns out, isn't hard to make either. The process is similar to making homemade almond or oat milk. Intimidating at first, but easy with practice. You simply soak the beans, remove the skins, blend with water, and then strain the milk through a cheesecloth so it's not grainy. No doubt, the few extra steps and equipment required, though minimal, puts off a lot of people, which is why Hodo sells not only soy milk and plain firm tofu, but also a whole line of pre-seasoned tofu cubes, crumbles, and burgers. Despite its versatility, and I would argue deliciousness, many of us are still confused to this day about tofu's origins, uses, and even healthfulness. That's where Tsai comes in: to remind us that many of the culinary treasures of our future may actually be found in our past.

———————

Like many prized foods, the discovery of tofu is cradled in legend. Tofu is thought to have been created by accident, when someone (some believe it was the scholar and philosopher Lord Liú Ān of of the Han dynasty) cooked soybeans and, instead of throwing out the excess liquid, flavored it with salt and vinegar, which curdled the mixture. That led to the first tofu-like substance, which, through trial and error, became the tofu we know today. It's possible to make a solid product from the milk or juice of any bean, but soybeans were cheap and omnipresent in Asia. Tofu making became a way to introduce variety and protein into the largely meatless diets of the ancient Chinese.

For those living in East Asia, tofu is a staple of daily life, similar to bread in the West. Like Tsai, many of those who grew up in China, Japan, Taiwan, or other East Asian countries have memories of buying freshly made tofu from a local market with their parents and grandparents. But for Westerners, it's still a relatively niche food associated with vegetarians and vegans. Its rising popularity in the United States can be attributed in part to *The Book of Tofu*, published in 1975, coauthored by William Shurtleff, an American, and his Japanese wife at the time, a chef named Akiko Aoyagi.

Tsai told me that Shurtleff still lives in the Bay Area, so I decided to pay him a visit. In his eighties, Shurtleff was remarkably sharp and agile, clearly a lifelong Zen practitioner. When I asked him about his life story, he paused and then answered, "The fundamental teaching of Buddhism is that everything changes. You have a name that doesn't change from the day you're born until the day you die, but that leads you to the perception that there is a continuing self." Fair enough, but the fact remains that Shurtleff devoted his life, or, as he would have it, his succession of lives, to learning and cataloging everything one could possibly know about the magic bean.

Shurtleff first came to Japan on an exchange program to learn about Zen Buddhism. He lived in a monastery for a few months, then decided to hitchhike across the country. When he returned to California to study at the legendary Tassajara Zen Center, his teacher urged him to go back to Japan to continue to learn the language and culture. There he met Aoyagi, a soy enthusiast who taught him how to prepare the foodstuff. Shurtleff was fascinated by tofu's affordability, versatility, and taste, and decided he wanted to bring tofu making to the West.

The couple began by approaching their local tofu maker in Japan, Aoyagi translating and Shurtleff taking copious notes and photographs to document every step of the process. They ended up visiting tofu masters all over the country, staying in Zen monasteries and eating with locals along the way. Although many of the masters were reluctant to share their wisdom at first—"Traditional tofu masters have a saying that there are two things they will not show another person: how to make babies and how to make tofu"—they found that the masters liked the idea of their knowledge being passed on to a Western audience.

Over a period of three years, the couple prepared more than a thousand tofu recipes and selected 250 for the book. Once it was complete, they embarked on a road trip across America to spread the tofu gospel. For four months in 1975, they taught people about the "bread of the East," as they called it, and apparently inspired several hundred Americans to open tofu shops across the country. When the couple moved to California, they set up the SoyInfo Center in Lafayette, just east of the Bay Area, where Shurtleff still lives, with a comprehensive library of the history of the foodstuff taking up the better part of his living room.

One of the most surprising things Shurtleff discovered when writing the book is that the United States was the leading producer of soy in the world, yet most Americans had never heard of tofu. That's because most of the soy grown in the U.S. wasn't being fed to humans, but to farmed animals. While cows naturally eat grass, chickens eat seeds and insects, and pigs are foraging animals that eat leaves, roots, and fruits, in the late nineteenth century, farmers began to feed soybean meal to their livestock, as it was cheap and, being protein-rich, fattened them up faster. After World War II, soy production began to climb even more, enabled by synthetic fertilizers and chemical pesticides. The USDA offered subsidies to corn and soy growers, guaranteeing income.

Since then, global soy production has exploded. It is thirteen times higher today than in the early 1960s and has more than doubled since the year 2000.[1] You might think that that's because a ton more people are eating soy foods like tofu, but more than three-quarters of global soy continues to be fed to livestock. Although farmers have been able to improve yields by growing more soy on the same amount of land, they have also expanded croplands, which has meant cutting down forests.[2]

These facts first entered the cultural consciousness with the publication of Frances Moore Lappé's classic *Diet for a Small Planet*, which was published just a few years before Shurtleff and Aoyagi's book. In 1971 Lappé wrote:

> Most people think of vegetarianism as an ethical stance against the killing of animals, unconventional, and certainly untraditional. But what I advocate is the return to the traditional diet on which our bodies evolved. Traditionally the human diet has centered on plant foods, with animal foods playing a supplementary role. Our digestive and metabolic system evolved over millions of years on such a diet. Only very recently have Americans, and people in some other industrial countries, begun to center their diets on meat. It is the meat-centered diet—and certainly the grain-fed-meat-centered diet—that is the fad.[3]

Just as Lappé said back in the '70s, the Oldways Project reminds us of the centrality of plants in diverse culinary heritages. Whether it's the

Mediterranean, Latin American, Asian, or African Heritage diets, they all advise eating leafy greens, legumes, vegetables, soy, whole grains, and herbs and spices, limiting fish or shellfish to two servings a week, having eggs and poultry only occasionally, and avoiding red meat and sweets.

Tsai may have grown up eating tofu and rice as part of his Asian heritage diet, but that specific combination is just one iteration of the grains-and-legumes power couple that forms the cornerstone of every ancestral diet. The types of grains and legumes consumed have varied by region—potatoes and quinoa in South America, corn in Central America, wheat in the Middle East and Europe, rice in Asia—yet no matter where we look around the world, entire populations have been sustained by starches. In China, the way people say hello is often by asking "Have you had your rice today?" And in some parts of Japan, instead of "How are you?" people ask, "Have you had enough *imo*?"—imo being a type of Japanese sweet potato known for its distinct sweetness.

When I first adopted a plant-based diet I worried, like everyone, that "carbs make you fat." But while processed carbohydrates like white flour surely impact your waistline, the complex carbohydrates found in whole foods such as starches keep us full longer as we convert the sugars into usable energy. A randomized control trial published in the prestigious *Nature Medicine* compared a "keto" (low-carb) diet with a low-fat (high-carb) healthful vegan diet. Even when the study participants on the vegan diet ate as much food as they wanted, they ate 700 fewer calories and burned more body fat, despite feeling completely satiated, compared to the keto subjects.[4] Turns out that we really do get fat from fat (and processed foods).

Dr. John McDougall learned this the hard way. Growing up he ate the Standard American Diet—meat, dairy, and eggs—until he had a massive stroke as an adolescent. The experience led him to become a doctor and, eventually, to discover the true diet of our ancestors. As a young doctor working in Hawaii, he was struck by a phenomenon he noticed in his patients, many of them of Asian descent: the children were far less healthy than their parents, who had grown up eating a lot of rice and vegetables, unlike their children, who embraced fast food.

That observation led him to conduct a comparative study of Japanese men living in Japan, Hawaii, and California. He found the lowest incidence of heart disease among men living in Japan, and the highest among men living in California (nearly 50 percent higher than in Hawaii). Men who moved to the United States increased their risk substantially.[5] Even more compelling evidence of the fact that diet and lifestyle matter more than genes is a study that showed a shared link of diabetes between dog and cat owners and their pets—if owners have type 2 diabetes, their pets are likely to as well.[6] "Diet and nutrition advice is often focused on how much we ought to eat and misses the point: More important than how much, how often, and when we eat, is what we eat," says Dr. McDougall. "We humans are built to thrive on starch. The more rice, corn, potatoes, sweet potatoes, and beans we eat, the trimmer, more energetic, and healthier we become. It's the food!"[7]

The ancient wisdom that starches are good for our health was rediscovered in the *National Geographic* Blue Zones project, which grew out of demographic work by Gianni Pes, an Italian doctor, and Michel Poulain, a French longevity expert, who identified Sardinia, Italy, as an epicenter of centenarians.[8] They partnered with Dan Buettner, a former explorer at *National Geographic*. Together, the team identified longevity hotspots—"Blue Zones"—around the world, including Ikaria, Greece; Nicoya, Costa Rica; Okinawa, Japan; and Loma Linda, California, home of the Seventh-day Adventists and the only Blue Zone in the United States.[9] In these regions, people eat a "plant slant" diet—as high as 85 percent of their calories from plant-based foods, especially lentils and beans such as fava, black, and soy. As the acclaimed nutritionist Marion Nestle writes, "Dietary patterns that best promote health derive most energy from plant foods, considerably less from foods of animal origin (meat, dairy, eggs), and even less from foods high in animal fats and sugar,"[10] and that is exactly how people in Blue Zones eat. They also engage in regular low-level exercise and other practices that promote connection and reduce stress.

Take Okinawa, Japan, where inhabitants have the world's longest life expectancy and suffer far less chronic diseases such as heart disease, breast and prostate cancers, and dementia. Dan Buettner learned of Okinawa from brothers Craig and Bradley Willcox. Together with Dr. Makoto Suzuki, the Japanese medical doctor who first discovered the longevity phenomenon, the trio popularized the community's ways of life in their book *The Okinawa Program*. In their research, they found that prior to WWII, more than half of the calories Okinawans consumed came from just one source—imo, which was introduced in the early seventeenth century and became a staple because it was one of the few things that grew reliably in the rocky soil. Nobody thinks it's a good idea to get all your calories from only one food source, but if you had to pick one, you could do a lot worse than the Japanese sweet potato. Imo is not only fat-free, but chock-full of flavonoids, vitamin C, fiber, and health-promoting carotenoids, making it one of the most healthful foods on the planet. It happens to be my favorite food.

With the help of *The Okinawa Program*'s research, Buettner and his team compared the macronutrient breakdown—the ratio of carbohydrates, fats, and protein—of the Okinawans before and after the war, when diets began to shift toward a Western model, and showed that meat and dairy represented only about 3 percent of their calories. A typical meal might consist of champuru (lightly stir-fried vegetables) with goya (bitter lemon), daikon (radish), okra, pumpkin, burdock root, and green papaya. Fish and meat served as the seasoning, rather than the main course—often on special occasions such as Lunar New Year—and dishes were prepared with an assortment of fresh herbs that were not only delicious but served medicinal purposes.

They also ate plenty of tofu. As both Minh Tsai and William Shurtleff told me, tofu for the Okinawans was (and is) what bread is in many cultures: a daily habit. Tofu is a source of flavonoids and lowers the risk of heart disease compared to meat, which raises both cholesterol and triglyceride levels. Overall, the plant-rich traditional Okinawan diet carries a low glycemic load, creates less inflammation and oxidative stress, and reduces risk for chronic age-related diseases.[11] The same is true for the other Blue Zones that Buettner and his team cataloged. In all the longevity hot spots, about four-fifths of the calories come from carbohydrate sources including vegetables, legumes, grains, potatoes, and fruits. The type of carbohydrate varies by region, with more grains eaten in Sardinia, Italy; more fruit in the Nicoya religion of Costa Rica; more greens and pasta in Ikaria, Greece; and more legumes and soy foods among the Seventh-day Adventists in Loma Linda, California.

But after the Second World War, dietary patterns shifted considerably. Within a generation, consumption of sweet potatoes in Okinawa dropped from 60 to less than 5 percent of the daily diet. Okinawans were understandably tired of eating imo for breakfast, lunch, and dinner for decades, and began to eat far more rice, bread, milk, meat, eggs, poultry, and Spam, a processed canned meat product given out by the American military. Within a generation, the island's landscape became dotted with American fast food joints like McDonald's, Burger King, and Taco Bell. While older generations in rural areas still follow a more traditional way of life, the new generation has embraced the Western diet.

There's a reason we often think of plant-based staples like rice, beans, and potatoes as "peasant food." As people become wealthier, they tend to abandon the foods eaten by their ancestors. As Marion Nestle observes, "Once people have access to meat, they usually do not return to eating plant-based diets unless they are forced to do so by economic reversal or are convinced to do so for reasons of religion, culture, or health."[12] Sadly, that shift shows up in their health outcomes, just as it did for the Okinawans, with people gaining weight and beginning to suffer from diet-related chronic conditions including heart disease and cancer.

Like many immigrant children, when he came to America, Tsai was excited to try all the fast food, but it got old quickly. "I started to miss the food of my homeland, the rituals in the kitchen, and I think maybe part of why I started my company is because it was a way to rediscover that heritage." I could relate. When we first immigrated to Canada, all I wanted was to be like the other children. I remember being excited to eat "normal food" at school, like Wonder Bread sandwiches with ham and cheese. But as I grew older, I suddenly longed for fresh dill, white potatoes, beets, pickles, borscht, and sauerkraut. I missed the fresh cucumbers and tomatoes my Babushka and Dedushka grew in our garden, and the jam they made from berries in the summer.

The American food landscape—perhaps as an analogy to its psyche—is characterized by extremes: "junk food" on the one hand and "health food" on the other. We eat a lot of hamburgers, hot dogs, milkshakes, and the like, which all include animal products. But we also think of ourselves as a "melting pot," thanks to our access to cuisines from all around the world. For inspiration, we need look no farther than our own richly diverse culinary histories and traditions, all of which derive from the colorful rainbow of plant foods. Better yet, we can combine them all and learn something new.

———

Back in Tsai's kitchen, it was time to put together our lunch. The tofu master pulled out some brown rice, as well as an array of steamed vegetables, including sweet potatoes, okra, asparagus, and artichoke hearts. "Just one more thing," he added, taking out a dish of what looked like tofu sheets marinating in some dark liquid. "This is yuba, and it's just been sitting in some soy sauce and a bit of sugar since this morning. I'm going to make you some mock duck." Tsai heated up some oil in a cast iron pan, and then added the yuba. Within minutes, it began to sizzle and smell remarkably like flesh.

When he finished, we each grabbed a clay bowl handmade by an Oakland-based ceramicist and served ourselves generous helpings of rice, veggies, and of course tofu, in three forms: the silken tofu with soy sauce, mock duck yuba, and an adobo-seasoned crumble that was about to join his array of pre-seasoned specialties. Rays of sun streamed into the kitchen, and I felt at home at his wooden kitchen table, remembering the times I'd cooked with my grandmother as a child.

We dug in, and I couldn't believe my taste buds. The bowl was prepared in a simple yet artful way, and each ingredient was as fresh as could be. I mentally cataloged each ingredient, promising myself that I would aim to cook like this at home more often. I am happy to say that I have kept my promise to myself, and since cooking with Tsai, tofu has become my new culinary love. I simply can't seem to get enough. Taking a few bites from his bowl, Tsai mused, "This is very much how we used to eat when I was a child in my family." The tofu master isn't vegan but eats primarily plants, and he explained that "Back home people couldn't afford a lot of meat, so it would mostly be used for flavor. We knew where everything comes from, and that was the norm."

While Bill Shurtleff's mission is to catalog the history of tofu, Minh Tsai's is restore its place as a staple of everyday life. Tsai is ensuring that the tofu he grew up with, and, even more important, the traditional way in which it is prepared and consumed, remains part of our culinary future, not only our past.

Conclusion

Trade-offs in the Future of Food

On Sunday mornings, you can find me at the Temescal farmers market, which borders Oakland and Berkeley in the East Bay. I'm there so often that my friends jokingly call it my "church," and honestly, the description isn't too far off. The pilgrimage begins with a bike ride from Lake Merritt up past Broadway, a major throughway that originates in Jack London Square, and travels north to where Telegraph and Claremont avenues intersect. The streets are unusually quiet in the early morning hours, until we begin to hear the buzz of vendors setting up for the day.

After we drop off our bikes, the first order of business is, predictably, coffee. We head to Rhetoric Coffee, where we order our once-a-week treat: a pair of almond milk lattés. Our friend James Parrish buys only the best-quality beans, sourced from farms where producers get paid more than fair trade minimums. The almond milk is from Beber, the stand next door, which sources its organic almonds from local California orchards. The two make for a dynamic duo: the deep and complex coffee flavor with the velvety smooth milk have converted me from a regular green tea drinker into an occasional coffee indulger.

Next, we stop at the Midwife and the Baker, owned by Jamie Shapiro (the midwife) and Mac McConnell (the baker), who like to say that their chosen professions are two of the oldest. McConnell has been teaching the art of bread making at the San Francisco Baking Institute since 2011. When the husband-and-wife team opened their own facility in 2015, they began to source their whole grain directly from California farmers and mill it fresh, rather than buying processed flour. You can taste the dedication in their fresh loaves, the aroma irresistible to market shoppers. Our favorites are the walnut currant and the sesame whole wheat, and we're usually done with half a loaf before we get home.

Then it's on to Tomatero Farm, which grows certified organic vegetables just a few miles inland from the California coast in Watsonville. The farm was founded by Adriana Silva and Chris Tuohig. In Spanish, *tomatero* means "tomato picker," and the farm was named by Silva's Nicaraguan grandmother, who chose the name when she learned that their first crop would be tomatoes. Their tomatoes are indeed sublime—sun-kissed burst-in-your-mouth goodness. Most of the workers on the farm are family members, and all employees are paid year-round wages above fair wage requirements. They also prioritize soil health, using plants, insects, and native hedgerows to increase soil fertility, and let the soil lie fallow to rejuvenate. Today they grow greens, broccoli, peppers, squash, melons, root vegetables, and, when they're in season, delectable strawberries, a special treat we look forward to every year.

We're regulars at the East Bay markets all year round, and our meals at home ebb and flow with the seasons. But they're always some combination of a grain, legume, seasonal vegetables, and a fresh dressing whipped up in the blender. In summer, I roast fresh corn and serve it on a bed of brown rice with pinto or black beans, lettuce, and tomato and red onion salsa, and garnish it with local avocado and lime and a flourish of cilantro. In autumn, I roast local squash with cinnamon and freshly ground black pepper and serve it on a bed of dino kale, sweet potatoes, Brussels sprouts, cauliflower, and parsnips with pomegranate, dates, and toasted pumpkin seeds in a garlicky tahini lemon dressing. In the winter months, I make a hearty potato leek soup with chard and collard greens along with fresh bread and parsley or a cashew cream mushroom risotto with balsamic reduction, tarragon, rosemary, and thyme. As winter turns once again to spring, I celebrate the warmer weather with a citrus salad of cara cara oranges, grapefruit, and tangelos alongside beets, asparagus, and fava beans. Nature provides us with an incredible array of colors, textures, and flavors, beckoning us to become curious about their endless possibilities.

I'd be the first to acknowledge my luck at settling down in the Bay Area, a place that, with its Mediterranean-like climate and year-round growing season, can only be described as a cornucopia. But I've been actively supporting farmers ever since I moved out of my parents' home, buying from farmers markets and signing up for community-supported agriculture (CSA) boxes wherever I could, including Boston, Paris, Nice, Berlin, Tel Aviv, New York, and Los Angeles. I always search for food cooperatives and shops that sell locally sourced produce, and often go out of my way to dine at farm-to-table restaurants. Living on a student budget for many years, I searched for the most affordable yet best quality produce I could find, always committed to paying a premium for food produced with intention and care.

As I sit at my desk and sip my favorite green tea (organically grown along the Li River in southeast China), musing on where the journey of this book has taken me, I'm tempted to say: Go to the farmers market, shop at co-ops and CSAs, dine at farm-to-table restaurants, find out how food gets on your plate along every step of the food chain, and of course, eat more plants. But as a sociologist, I know that solutions cannot merely boil down to changing the practices of individual consumers. Our food choices are dictated by far more than our idiosyncratic tastes and preferences.

The truth is that food has historically hardly ever been a matter of individual choice. Not so long ago, people only ate food that was available where they lived. We ate in season, and we certainly didn't eat meat three times a day. Most of our calories came from plant staples such as rice in Asia, potatoes in South America, corn in Central America, cassava and yams in Africa, wheat in Europe, and a variety of heritage beans and legumes, along with whatever vegetables, fungi, and fruits happened to be in season.

In other words, plants, not animals, have been the main source of calories and nutrients for humanity, coevolving with our species. Even today, the longest-living populations around the world have a "plant slant"—that is, the vast majority of their calories come from plants. Despite what advocates of "paleo" or "keto" diets may claim, animal protein took on critical importance in our evolutionary history in part because of its scarcity. In nearly every culture, meat held a high status precisely because it was considered a luxury, unlike the commonplace yet indispensable plant foods on which we relied for survival.

All that changed with the advent of the Agricultural Revolution, when we domesticated animals and consumed their flesh and other by-products more frequently, especially in colder climates. Since the Industrial Revolution, animal products have accounted for a greater proportion of our diet than ever before in human history. In fact, humans and livestock account for nearly all of the biomass on earth.[1] We, and the animals we raise for food, now make up most of the hungry eaters straining natural resources. Most of the wild animals have been killed off. Our desire for cheap and omnipresent meat means that we are literally crowding out all the other species in existence.

For most of our history, the biggest problem to solve around food was its shortage. But now, especially in the West, we are overproducing food, only to cycle much of it back through farmed animals, while hunger continues to plague most of humanity. Somehow, we still think that, as the old advertisement goes, the answer to the question "What's for dinner?" should be "Beef." Worse still, while there is growing interest in plant-based diets in the Western world, the average amount of meat consumed per person globally has nearly doubled in the past fifty years, outpacing population growth.[2]

Projections show that to avert environmental disaster by 2050, we need to reduce our meat consumption by at least a third, and by half in North

America and Europe, the continents that consume the most by far. But many people still eat eggs for breakfast and yogurt as a snack, put dairy milk in their coffee, add a slice of ham to their sandwich for lunch, and choose a piece of meat or fish for dinner, all in one day. A reduction from that daily menu to a couple of eggs and a small piece of meat or fish once a week seems like a hefty drop, yet that is how humanity has eaten for most of our natural history.

Even as many nations claim to be taking measures to reduce carbon footprints, their governments still heavily subsidize animal products, supporting the animal agriculture industry rather than public health and our planet. It's no surprise that we are now seeing an attempt by the private sector to take the lead. Innovative companies are crafting clever technologies—cell-cultured and plant-based meat, ocean farming, indoor vertical farming, and even industrial-scale insect production— which they promise will fix the problems in our food system. Yet as innovative as these technologies may be, we must consider them from the perspective of an entire food system, which includes their inevitable downsides.

If there's one takeaway from this book, it's that no matter which food system we choose, trade-offs are inevitable. If we embrace the techno-optimistic "protein transition" envisioned by Bruce Friedrich and others, we will potentially save the lives of billions of sentient beings. But we will also contend with products made in our current commodity crop system, in which crops are grown with chemical fertilizers, sprayed with herbicides, and then heavily processed. These foods are certainly a win for animals, which in my view means they cannot be rejected outright. But they do not represent as radical a shift in the food system as they might claim.

On the other hand, if we embrace Emma Jagoz's vision of regenerative agriculture, we may get closer to what many people believe to be the ideal way to eat, but we will face the age-old challenges of farmers: the constraints of the growing season and the difficulty of scaling a labor-intensive operation. Not surprisingly, regeneratively grown food is out of reach for many people. But the rising interest in urban and suburban farming, which is how Moon Valley Farm got its start, shows us that more people are keen on producing healthful food for their communities, and supporting their efforts will go a long way to recreating the tapestry of local food producers that used to feed us all.

The tension between the futurists and the traditionalists in the vegan movement is especially poignant around the issue of acquisitions: industry incumbents buying out small mission-driven brands. Many vegans, for example, commend the Tysons, Cargills, and Danones for embracing the plant-based revolution. They see acquisitions by industry incumbents as a boon to small mission-driven companies, giving them better access to capital and distribution channels while reducing their competition. Consider the case of plant-based milk, which became omnipresent in coffee shops and grocery stores after companies such as Silk and So Delicious were acquired by Danone.

But others see these developments as a threat. One vocal critic of corporate dominance in the "alternative protein" sector is Philip H. Howard, a professor at Michigan State University.[3] Howard's concern is that meat and dairy companies' efforts to reframe themselves as "protein companies" obfuscates their intentions to continue business as usual. He believes that the excitement around novel food technologies "disrupting" the food system misses the point that most alternative protein products do not represent a meaningful transition away from our agro-industrial complex.

It's true that a "protein" transition doesn't address some of the bigger issues in our food system. One of these is that if we move away from animal agriculture, many of those at the bottom of the hierarchy—underpaid slaughterhouse workers (many of them undocumented) and farmers raising poultry and pigs for large conglomerates—will be left without jobs.[4] Recognizing these problems, a few prominent vegan activists—most notably the Transfarmation Project founded by Mercy for Animals—are working to help animal farmers switch to growing plant crops (miraculously, hemp and mushrooms require similar conditions to chickens). We need far more of these kinds of creative solutions.

We also need food technology companies to take responsibility for how their products are sourced, produced, and distributed, improving the system as a whole along the entire food chain. The food scholar Garrett Broad calls solutions that combine technology with social concern "food tech justice,"[5] whose basic question is "How can novel food technologies be used to uplift communities, rather than solely the profits of companies?"

As the political economist Jan Dutkiewicz has written, governments must play a role. Instead of propping up an agricultural industry that harms animals, pollutes our environment, and causes public health issues, it should cut back on subsidies and help farmers transition away from monocultures of soy, wheat, and corn. If we were to grow leguminous crops domestically, for example, we could not only support more healthful plant-based products but perhaps even grow feedstock for cell-cultured meat, creating blended or hybrid products that require less animal input. Regulation should also protect consumers from "greenwashing," false and exaggerated label claims about their environmental and health impacts such as "pasture-raised," "wild-caught," or "humanely treated," which are often misleading.

I think it's possible for the techno-optimist and regenerative visions to coexist, but only if they recognize their common enemy—factory farming—and the enduring problems of industrialization. Instead of reinforcing false dichotomies, why not work together to brainstorm about how to weave regenerative farming practices into the techno-optimistic futures of food? Likewise, let's work together to avoid falling into the trap of agrarian fantasies that have little to do with the reality of what it takes to feed a growing population. Whatever solutions we come up with, we should always remember that innovation must be used to truly transform, not simply "disrupt," the most important system humanity has ever cultivated.

———

Even if everyone agreed on a shared vision for a more sustainable food system, there are still many barriers to overcome. Unlike biological (diseases) or social (memes) phenomena, veganism is a case of what's known in social science as "complex contagion." It's complex in that it's a set of behaviors that is hard to reinforce. In other words, hearing about veganism isn't enough to get someone invested, even if they learn about the benefits of the lifestyle. In fact, with complex behavior change, it takes networks of people to reinforce it, including friends, family, coworkers, and the broader community.

As an "early adopter" of veganism, I am still in the vast minority of society. There are surveys suggesting that vegans are more socially stigmatized than immigrants, atheists, and asexuals. Only drug addicts are seen more negatively.[6] Vegans are also the least favorably evaluated group among those who choose alternative lifestyles due to health (lactose intolerants and those who avoid gluten due to celiac disease) or religious reasons (kosher or halal).[7] In fact, among people curious about the lifestyle, "vegaphobia" is the chief obstacle.[8] No wonder that research finds that applying the "vegan" label to meal options actually lowers their appeal.[9]

There's also the problem of "selection bias." Vegans can be self-righteous about their moral beliefs, even smug. Who hasn't heard the old joke, "How do you recognize a vegan at a dinner party? Don't worry—they'll tell you!" Many ardent vegans joined the cause after exposure to footage of grotesque cruelty to animals. They assume that because these tactics worked on them, they will work on everyone else. But many people are turned off by graphic videos, and coming off as being on a moral high horse is often not the best way to inspire others.

I can understand why, for many people, a vegan lifestyle seems unappealing, overwhelming, or even downright offensive. As we know, meat has played a key part in our cultural and evolutionary history, and habits are notoriously difficult to break. Veganism requires a shift in identity as well as the embrace of a social category still on the fringe. Even when people do try a vegan lifestyle, the "relapse rate" is as high as 70 percent.[10] This is partly because being vegan in a nonvegan world is hard, but also because the vegan movement places an emphasis on moral perfection. Yet, as we have seen, long-lasting, sustainable change doesn't come from a place of shame, judgment, and guilt. It comes from a place of joy and a sense of belonging.

One of the things that gives me hope for the plight of animals is that speciesism—the idea that humans are inherently superior to nonhuman animals—isn't as baked into us as we might expect. Lucius Caviola, a brilliant psychologist and friend I met at Harvard (he's now at Oxford University), has done pioneering experimental work on speciesism and found that it is socially reinforced with age. One of his most fascinating studies compares children's and adults' attitudes toward nonhuman animals and shows that when young children (five to nine years old) are asked who should be saved among different numbers of humans and animals, they show a weaker tendency to prioritize humans. Children choose to save multiple dogs over one human, and even multiple pigs (although they value dogs more than pigs), while adults routinely choose to save one human over even a hundred dogs or pigs.

We can argue all day about the moral calculus involved in assessing the equivalence of human and nonhuman animal lives, but Caviola's research reveals that these beliefs are not entirely innate. His work suggests that speciesism is at least in part socially shaped and could conceivably be reversed. Many other intuitions humans have had throughout history—the earth is flat, men are superior to women, certain "races" are more intelligent than others, homosexuality is a sin, and so on—have at best been found to be false, and at worst led to unfathomable historical tragedies.

My view is that such a tragedy is unfolding in our midst. I believe that the treatment of nonhuman animals is the last socially acceptable moral atrocity. Every single day, *billions* of land animals and *trillions* of aquatic creatures are raised and slaughtered for food. Even though most people say they don't want animals to suffer—and they say so sincerely—there is a disconnect between the affection they feel for their pets and the animals who suffer on factory farms every day to sustain our gustatory desires.

Fortunately, we already see signs of the tide changing. Not only are there more people embracing a vegan lifestyle, but moral regard toward animals is changing too. It began with companion animals and horses in the nineteenth century, alongside the vegetarian movement, and has grown with the vegan and animal rights movements in the twentieth century. Today, it is practically socially unacceptable to wear real fur, something omnipresent until the 2000s. In state after state, those working on behalf of animal welfare are winning battles large and small on behalf of those with no voice to represent themselves in our courts of law.

We also see some governments stepping in and taking drastic measures to reverse the tide of climate change and biodiversity loss. In 1996 for example, the Costa Rican government restricted logging to incentivize landowners to conserve and encourage reforestation of land that had been converted to pasture. Within two decades, they doubled the size of their tropical rainforests, increased jobs, and reduced the livestock industry by one-third. Plus, their economy improved, rather than suffered, as many in the animal industry would like us to believe.[11]

There's also the fact that lasting social change happens, not as we might expect, from the top down, but instead from the bottom up. The work of my husband, Douglas Guilbeault (he's a network scholar), shows that when it comes to spreading new and sometimes controversial ideas—changes in diet, exercise routines, political leanings, or attitudes about new technologies—it is actually the people on the fringe who are often most important, not the influencers.[12] So the more that people meet, talk to, and most important, eat with others, the more the zeitgeist will shift.

While widespread veganism may not be inevitable, by the time our great-grandchildren are born, I hope they will be surprised to learn that we used to consume animals at such scale. Our own great-grandparents would be amazed to hear that we eat meat for breakfast, lunch, and dinner without a second thought about how it got to our table. Time and time again, history has shown the expansion of a moral circle that increasingly includes more individuals. But which path, exactly, will lead to the moral circle expanding to encompass all nonhuman animals remains to be seen.

———

Is there one ethical way to eat? The short answer is, probably not. But the longer answer is that this was the wrong question all along.

For me, grappling with the trade-offs inherent in any of the solutions offered to fix our broken food system has been a long and, admittedly, painful process of trying to reconcile conflicting versions of reality. It took a long time for me to realize that this struggle is the true journey that I have been on with this book. When at last I embraced the ambiguities and let go of my assumptions about finding the "right answer," I was able to step into a place where, as the Buddhists might say, I could hold multiple realities in the palms of my hands. A book that I thought would be about veganism turned out to be about the much larger quest of discovering what kind of food system I wanted to build, and how.

In the end, I still believe that a healthy and intentional vegan lifestyle is by far the most ethical way I have found to live. As the Oxford scientists Joseph Poore and Thomas Nemecek say in their blockbuster *Science* paper, "a vegan diet is probably the single biggest way to reduce your impact on planet Earth, not only greenhouse gases, but global acidification, eutrophication, land use, and water use."[13] But now I believe that instead of being the endpoint, veganism should be the starting point toward a lifestyle not only concerned with the fate of other animals, but also the human and environmental ethics of food.

Our individual choices are undoubtedly a drop in the bucket and yet, they matter. Some of our life choices seem much more consequential than others—switching careers, getting married, or having a child will most certainly have a profound impact on your life. Other choices, like what to wear on a certain day or what to eat for breakfast, don't seem nearly as consequential. But when we look closer, we observe that those seemingly mundane everyday choices aggregate into the unimaginably large and complex systems in which we are embedded every day. We must remember, though, that those systems only exist because each day we make choices that reinforce them, and together, we can shift the needle to another system altogether.

Don't forget that even if veganism seems too difficult, significant harm reduction is still within reach. Simply by virtue of living in an industrialized and wealthy country, we have the power—and I would argue the moral obligation—to change our behavior for the better, and it is okay to start small. Choose oat milk for your coffee, eat a vegan breakfast each day, or eat only vegan at home. If you would have told me I'd be vegan while I was still living in the south of France enjoying all the brie, croissants, and gelato as before, I would never have believed you, and yet here I am, nearly a decade later.

Does this mean that I believe my diet is ethically perfect? Certainly not. Many issues remain with plant-based diets that rely heavily on products like almond milk (almonds are water-intensive, though much less so than dairy);[14] avocadoes, which are often farmed in places with gang exploitation; or berries, bananas, and mangoes grown halfway across the world and transported, out of season, in large shipping containers on freighters and trucks that run on fossil fuels. I make a point of not eating berries out of season and avoiding tropical fruits unless I happen to be in a place where they are locally grown, but I can't always find organic food when I travel, so I do the best I can. These decisions, though small, still go a long way toward eating a more ethical, culturally sensitive, and sustainable diet.

For me, ignorance is no longer blissful. Bliss now comes from the knowledge that my food has been grown in a system that supports regeneration and a better future for generations to come. It comes from getting to know the farmers in my community, feasting with friends on meals I cooked from scratch, and sharing in the joy of nourishing food knowing that I am contributing not only to my own well-being, but that of those around me, humans, nonhumans, and the planet, as best I am able.

People often ask me whether my choice to embrace veganism ever feels like a sacrifice. "But don't you miss *cheese*?" they ask, a look of utter disbelief on their faces. "How is your energy level? Are you sure you're getting enough protein? You must make exceptions when you're traveling, right?" In fact, I feel that the decision to choose a vegan lifestyle is the best one I've ever made, and my only regret is not having done it sooner. That's because for me, and for many of the fellow vegans I've come to meet over nearly a decade traveling around the world, that choice is rarely about what I'm giving up, but about what I'm gaining, on a personal, societal, and global level. Most profoundly, I've discovered that the choice to be vegan every day has led to an existential sigh of relief that comes from knowing that I am living in alignment with my own values.

The environmentalist David Attenborough refers to the film *A Life on Our Planet* as his "witness statement." Let this book be my witness statement to the kind of food system I hope we have the courage, tenacity, and dedication to build together. To do so, we must all embark on an inner journey to discover what part we might play in that larger whole. Albert Einstein, himself a vegetarian, once wrote to a friend in a letter:

> A human being is a part of the whole, called by us "Universe," a part limited in time and space. We experience our thoughts and feelings as something separated from the rest—a kind of optical delusion of his consciousness. This delusion is a kind of prison for us, restricting us to our personal desires and to affection for a few persons nearest to us. Our task must be to free ourselves from this prison by widening our circle of compassion to embrace all living creatures and the whole nature in its beauty. Nobody is able to achieve this completely, but the striving for such achievement is in itself a part of the liberation and a foundation for inner security.[15]

Aside from the air we breathe, there is no better reminder of the interconnectedness of all things than the food we eat. Each forkful makes us who we are, literally and figuratively. This book, and the many years that went into my graduate work before it, has been my meditation on what a just and healthful future of food could look like, and the definitive role of plants—and our own diverse culinary histories—in building a food system that is more nourishing for all. So next time you ask yourself "What shall I eat today?"—remember that what you're really asking is "What kind of world do I want to live in?"

ACKNOWLEDGMENTS

We often hear it takes a village to raise a child. While I have not yet raised a child, I know it takes an entire community to bring a book to life: from initial conception and germination, through the inevitably difficult labor, to the miraculous birth, and at last, the moment it takes its place in the world.

The initial seeds of this book were planted over a decade ago while I was a graduate student at Harvard University in search of a dissertation topic. I am deeply grateful to my brilliant advisors Michèle Lamont, Bart Bonikowski, and Vanina Leschziner for shaping my intellectual trajectory. Your emphasis on rigor and objectivity formed the solid scientific foundation on which this book is based. I owe deep thanks to Lorne Tepperman, my mentor for the last two decades, not only for your confidence in me, but for your humor, friendship, and love.

I am humbled and awed to be surrounded by a pantheon of mentors I admire in the world of intentional eating. I am deeply grateful for the guidance of Michael Pollan, whose ideas have captured my imagination for my entire career. Your curiosity about our place in the natural world—and its relationships to us—has inspired me both professionally and personally. I am thankful for your presence in my life, and to you and Judith Belzer for welcoming us into your home. Beginning and ending this book at your desk felt like meaningful bookends for this project.

I am grateful to Will Rosenzweig for your meditations on gardening as a lived metaphor, for the many seeds you planted in my mind, and for quoting Rainer Maria Rilke during a bout of writer's block. Your students and mentees are fortunate to have you in their lives. I am grateful to Naomi Starkman, not only for your brilliance, but your warmth, generosity, and for teaching me to garden. You are a gift to all who know you.

I am honored to work with my entire book team. First and foremost, this book would not exist without "word nerd" Margo Beth Fleming, the book midwife who saw an author within me before I truly could. There is no better guide to the literary world, and your advice has been essential at every single step of the entire labor. Thank you for reading me, and for reading so many others I admire.

I am grateful for the incredible team at Bloomsbury who gave this book a home. Ben Hyman, your thoughtfulness and trust in my voice grounded me as my writing developed. Morgan Jones, your enthusiasm and dedication during the editing stage truly made my ideas far more readable and digestible. I am thankful for Akshaya Iyer, Marie Coolman, Lauren Ollerhead, and Lauren Moseley for helping me to bring this book from my desk to its readers.

I am grateful to all who agreed to be featured in this book, welcoming me into their kitchens and their worlds. Thank you to Bruce Friedrich, Ethan Brown, Miyoko Schinner, Aryé Elfenbein, Justin Kolbeck, Frohman Anderson, Chris Kerr, Lisa Feria, Matthew Hayek, Michael Pollan, Emma Jagoz, T. Colin Campbell, Dean Ornish, Matthew Kenney, Dick Gregory, Bryant Terry, Bill Shurtleff, and Minh Tsai. I owe tribute to pioneer Donald Watson, who coined the term "vegan" and inspired the title of this book. Your collective dedication to find a more just and sustainable way to feed our world moves me.

I am humbled by the people who endorsed and helped to promote this book—thank you for elevating my voice. For their thought partnership, I am grateful to Matthew Hayek, Max Bazerman, Jan Dutkiewicz, Dave Mackey, Chen Cohen, Matteo de Vos, and Rasa. I am grateful to the magical Noreen Fukumori for designing the "Good Eater Food Pyramid." I am enormously grateful for the support of my patrons, who wake up each day dedicated to selflessly saving as many animal lives as possible.

It isn't easy being vegan, but it is far easier when you are surrounded by incredible vegan friends. I am grateful to my sociologist francophile yogi doppelgänger Lauren Valentino, forever my mirror. I am grateful to Samantha Derrick, my vegan twin and the Yang to my Yin. I am thankful for my vegan moai and "Build It" team Tara Kemp and Robby Barbaro, who inspire me each day. I am grateful to my former student and friend Grace Roberts Burbank for being an early reader.

I am beyond grateful for my cherished soul tribe for your light and love: Danielle Flores, Olesia Bissett, Brian Spears, Scott Blew, Raman Frey, Karin Johnson, and Sebastien Bicard. I am grateful to Jon Rubenstein and Karin Swann-Rubenstein for your generosity, vulnerability, and strength. For their empathy and wisdom, and I am grateful for the loving support of Jed Bickford, Gal Szekely, and Kristina Baré.

I am grateful for the communities I have cultivated in the Bay Area. First, my team at Plant Futures, who dedicate each day to growing a meaningful movement: Samantha Derrick, Brittany Sartor, Cynthia Bazán, Grace Roberts Burbank, Eric Sirvinskas, Chema Padilla, Will Rosenzweig, and of course, our entire community. I am grateful to my Berkeley family: my studio mates at Moonflower Studio, my "village" at the Hidden Café, my friends at the Green Yogi, and to all the farmers who nourish us each week. I am grateful to my communities in San Francisco, at The Commons and The Center, mind and heart of the city.

I would like to thank a few other lifelong companions. Cesaria Evora, the "barefoot diva" from Cape Verde, whose voice uplifts my soul. The poet Diego Perez, a friend to my authentic self, and the voice of our healing generation. Finally, the Mesa Refuge, a writing residency perched on the edge of Point Reyes where I finished the manuscript of this book. It is a mystical place where one can, as the Irish poet John O'Donohue remarks, be part of the "ancient conversation between the ocean and the land."

At last, I am grateful for my family—Galina Gheihman, Boris Gheihman, and Natalia Sutova, whose love and support fills my heart, and for their willingness to become good eaters. To my grandparents, Svetlana Sutova and Serghei Sutov, who are with me always. I am grateful for the loving embrace of my husband's family. Deepest of all, I am grateful for my "ineffabond" with Douglas Guilbeault, in whom I have found not only a life partner, but a spiritual sanctuary. At last, I am grateful to you, the reader, for thinking alongside me about how we can cultivate a more equitable, just, and nourishing food system for all.

NOTES

INTRODUCTION

1. Good Food Institute, "2020 State of the Industry Report: Plant-Based Meat, Eggs, and Dairy," https://gfi.org/wp-content/uploads/2021/05/COR-SOTIR -Plant-based-meat-eggs-and-dairy-2021-0504.pdf.

2. Good Food Institute, "2021 U.S. Retail Market Insights for the Plant-Based Industry," https://gfi.org/marketresearch/.

3. Meticulous Research, "Plant Based Food Market by Type," August 2022, https://www.meticulousresearch.com/product/plant-based-food-market-5108.

4. Good Food Institute, "2021 U.S. Retail Market Insights."

5. Jeffrey M. Jones, "In U.S., 4% Identify as Vegetarian, 1% as Vegan," Gallup, August 24, 2023, https://news.gallup.com/poll/510038/identify-vegetarian -vegan.aspx.

6. Justin McCarthy and Scott DeKoster, "Nearly One in Four in U.S. Have Cut Back on Eating Meat," Gallup, January 27, 2020, https://news.gallup.com/poll /282779/nearly-one-four-cut-back-eating-meat.aspx.

7. Smart Protein, "Plant-Based Foods in Europe: What Do Consumers Want?" 2021, https://smartproteinproject.eu/consumer-attitudes-plant-based-food -report/.

8. Tao Huang, Bin Yang, Jusheng Zheng, Guipu Li, Mark L. Wahlqvist, and Duo Li, "Cardiovascular Disease Mortality and Cancer Incidence in Vegetarians:

A Meta-Analysis and Systematic Review," *Annals of Nutrition and Metabolism* 60, no. 4 (2012): 233–40, https://pubmed.ncbi.nlm.nih.gov/22677895/.

9. Rami S. Najjar and Rafaela G. Feresin, "Plant-Based Diets in the Reduction of Body Fat: Physiological Effects and Biochemical Insights," *Nutrients* 11, no. 11 (2019): 2712, https://pubmed.ncbi.nlm.nih.gov/31717463/.

10. Jenny Chang-Claude, Silke Hermann, Ursula Eilber, and Karen Steindorf, "Lifestyle Determinants and Mortality in German Vegetarians and Health-Conscious Persons: Results of a 21-Year Follow-Up," *Cancer Epidemiology and Prevention Biomarkers* 14, no. 4 (2005): 963–68, https://pubmed.ncbi.nlm.nih.gov/15824171/.

11. Dan Buettner and Sam Skemp, "Blue Zones: Lessons from the World's Longest Lived," *American Journal of Lifestyle Medicine* 10, no. 5 (2016): 318–21, https://pubmed.ncbi.nlm.nih.gov/30202288/.

12. Preetha Anand et al., "Cancer Is a Preventable Disease That Requires Major Lifestyle Changes," *Pharmaceutical Research* 25, no. 9 (2008): 2097–116, https://pubmed.ncbi.nlm.nih.gov/18626751/.

13. Walter C. Willett, "Diet and Cancer," *Oncologist* 5, no. 5 (2000): 393–404, https://pubmed.ncbi.nlm.nih.gov/11040276/.

14. Monica Dinu, Rosanna Abbate, Gian F. Gensini, Alessandro Casini, and Francesco Sofi, "Vegetarian, Vegan Diets and Multiple Health Outcomes: A Systematic Review with Meta-Analysis of Observational Studies," *Critical Reviews in Food Science and Nutrition* 57, no. 17 (2017): 3640–49, https://pubmed.ncbi.nlm.nih.gov/26853923/.

15. WHO Team, "Cancer: Carcinogenicity of the Consumption of Red Meat and Processed Meat," WHO Newsroom, October 26, 2015, https://who.int/news-room/questions-and-answers/item/cancer-carcinogenicity-of-the-consumption-of-red-meat-and-processed-meat.

16. IARC Working Group on the Evaluation of Carcinogenic Risks to Humans, "Red Meat and Processed Meat: Volume 114. IARC Monographs on the Evaluation of Carcinogenic Risks to Humans," World Health Organization, Geneva; International Agency for Research on Cancer, Lyon, 2018, https://publications

.iarc.fr/Book-And-Report-Series/Iarc-Monographs-On-The-Identification
-Of-Carcinogenic-Hazards-To-Humans/Red-Meat-And-Processed-Meat
-2018.

17. Wei Lu, Hanwen Chen, Yuequn Niu, Han Wu, Dajing Xia, and Yihua Wu,
"Dairy Products Intake and Cancer Mortality Risk: A Meta-Analysis of 11
Population-Based Cohort Studies," *Nutrition Journal* 15, no. 1 (2016): 91, https://
pubmed.ncbi.nlm.nih.gov/27765039/.

18. Sean Harrison et al., "Does Milk Intake Promote Prostate Cancer Initiation
or Progression via Effects on Insulin-Like Growth Factors (IGFs)? A Systematic Review and Meta-Analysis," *Cancer Causes and Control* 28, no. 6 (2017):
497–528, https://pubmed.ncbi.nlm.nih.gov/28361446/.

19. N. E. Allen, P. N. Appleby, G. K. Davey, and T. J. Key, "Hormones and Diet:
Low Insulin-Like Growth Factor-I but Normal Bioavailable Androgens in
Vegan Men," *British Journal of Cancer* 83, no. 1 (2000): 95–97, https://pubmed
.ncbi.nlm.nih.gov/10883675/.

20. Christopher Doering, "Where the Dollars Go: Lobbying a Big Business for
Large Food and Beverage CPGs," *FoodDive*, December 6, 2021, https://fooddive
.com/news/where-the-dollars-go-lobbying-a-big-business-for-large-food
-and-beverage-c

21. Olivier J. Wouters, "Lobbying Expenditures and Campaign Contributions by
the Pharmaceutical and Health Product Industry in the United States, 1999–
2018," *JAMA Internal Medicine* 180, no. 5 (2020): 1–10, https://www.ncbi.nlm
.nih.gov/pmc/articles/PMC7054854/.

22. David L. Katz, "Plant-Based Diets for Reversing Disease and Saving the Planet:
Past, Present, and Future," *Advances in Nutrition* 10, no. 4 (2019), S304–307,
https://pubmed.ncbi.nlm.nih.gov/31728489/.

23. The Editors, "To Fight Antimicrobial Resistance, Start with Farm Animals,"
Scientific American, March 1, 2023, https://scientificamerican.com/article
/to-fight-antimicrobial-resistance-start-with-farm-animals/.

24. Institute for Health Metrics and Evaluation, "Global Burden of Disease
(GBD)," 2019, https://healthdata.org/research-analysis/gbd.

CHAPTER ONE: SETTING THE TABLE

1. The Vegan Society, "Ripened by Human Determination: 70 Years of The Vegan Society," *The Vegan Society*, 2014, downloadable pdf available at https://www .vegansociety.com/sites/default/files/uploads/Ripened%20by%20human%20 determination.pdf.

2. The Vegan Society, "Definition of Veganism," *The Vegan Society*, 2022, https://vegansociety.com/go-vegan/definition-veganism.

3. Ibid.

4. George J. Armelagos, "Brain Evolution, the Determinates of Food Choice, and the Omnivore's Dilemma," *Critical Reviews in Food Science and Nutrition* 54, no. 10 (2014): 1330–41, https://pubmed.ncbi.nlm.nih.gov/24564590/.

5. Colin Barras, "Ancient Leftovers Show the Real Paleo Diet Was a Veggie Feast," *New Scientist*, December 5, 2016, https://newscientist.com/article/2115127 -ancient-leftovers-show-the-real-paleo-diet-was-a-veggie-feast/.

6. Bethany L. Turner and Amanda L. Thompson, "Beyond the Paleolithic Prescription: Incorporating Diversity and Flexibility in the Study of Human Diet Evolution," *Nutrition Reviews* 71, no. 8 (2013): 501–10, https://pubmed.ncbi .nlm.nih.gov/23865796/.

7. Richard Wrangham, "The Evolution of Human Nutrition," *Current Biology* 23, no. 9 (2013): R354–55, https://pubmed.ncbi.nlm.nih.gov/23660356/.

8. Julio Mercader, "Mozambican Grass Seed Consumption During the Middle Stone Age," *Science* 326, no. 5960 (2009):1680–83, https://pubmed.ncbi.nlm.nih .gov/20019285/.

9. Colin Spencer, *The Heretic's Feast: A History of Vegetarianism* (London: Fourth Estate, 1993), xi.

10. Walter Isaacson, *Leonardo da Vinci* (New York: Simon & Schuster, 2017), 130.

11. Ibid.

12. Rosamund Bartlett, *Tolstoy: A Russian Life* (Boston: Houghton Mifflin Harcourt, 2011).

13. Nico Slate, *Gandhi's Search for the Perfect Diet* (Seattle: University of Washington Press, 2019), 51.

14. Ibid., 64.

15. Ibid., 46.

16. William Shurtleff and Akiko Aoyagi, "Loma Linda Foods: Work with Soyfoods," SoyInfo Center, 2004, https://soyinfocenter.com/HSS/loma_linda_foods.php.

17. William Shurtleff and Akiko Aoyagi, "History of Meat Alternatives (960 CE to 2014)," SoyInfo Center, 2014, https://www.soyinfocenter.com/books/179.

18. Natasha Ishak, "How William Pester Pioneered the Hippie Lifestyle in California in the 1910s," *All That's Interesting*, June 18, 2020, https://allthatsinteresting.com/william-pester.

19. Jonathan Kauffman, *Hippie Food: How Back-to-the-Landers, Longhairs, and Revolutionaries Changed the Way We Eat* (New York: HarperCollins, 2019), 28.

20. James Jasper and Dorothy Nelkin, *The Animal Rights Crusade: The Growth of a Moral Protest* (New York: Free Press, 1992).

21. Stanford Encyclopedia of Philosophy, 2015, "Jeremy Bentham," https://plato.stanford.edu/entries/bentham/.

22. Peter Singer, *Animal Liberation* (New York: HarperCollins, 1975), 8.

23. Lucius Caviola, Jim A. C. Everett, and Nicola Faber, "The Moral Standing of Animals: Towards a Psychology of Speciesism," *Journal of Personal Social Psychology* 116, no. 6 (2019): 1011–29, https://pubmed.ncbi.nlm.nih.gov/29517258/.

24. Food and Agriculture Organization of the United Nations (FAO), 2020, https://fao.org/faostat/en/?#data/.

25. Rebecca Ackerman, "Inside Effective Altruism, Where the Far Future Counts a Lot More than the Present," *MIT Technology Review*, October 17, 2022, https://technologyreview.com/2022/10/17/1060967/effective-altruism-growth/.

26. ALF, 2023, "The ALF Credo and Guidelines," *AnimalsLiberationFront.com*, October 15, 2023, https://www.abolitionistapproach.com/media/links/p2360/animal-liberation.pdf.

27. PETA, 1984, *Unnecessary Fuss*, https://peta.org/videos/unnecessary-fuss/.

CHAPTER TWO: PARADIGM SHIFT

1. Matt Ball and Bruce Friedrich, *The Animal Activist's Handbook: Maximizing Our Positive Impact in Today's World* (New York: Lantern Books, 2008), xiii.

2. Ibid., 7.

3. Ibid., *Animal Activist's Handbook*, 5.

4. Everett M. Rogers, *Diffusion of Innovations* (New York: Free Press, 2003).

5. Bloomberg, "'Beef Will Always Be King.' Americans Are Set to Eat More Meat in 2018 than Ever Before," *Fortune*, January 2, 2018, https://fortune.com/2018 /01/02/meat-consumption-america-2018/.

6. Brock Bastian, Steve Loughnan, Nick Haslam, and Helena R. M. Radke, "Don't Mind Meat? The Denial of Mind to Animals Used for Human Consumption," *Personality and Social Psychology Bulletin* 38, no. 2 (2012): 247–56, https://pubmed.ncbi.nlm.nih.gov/21980158/.

7. Melanie Joy, *Why We Love Dogs, Eat Pigs, and Wear Cows: An Introduction to Carnism* (Newburyport, MA: Red Wheel, 2011).

8. Oleschuk, Merin, Josée Johnston, and Shyon Baumann, "Maintaining Meat: Cultural Repertoires and the Meat Paradox in a Diverse Sociocultural Context," *Sociological Forum* 32, no. 2 (2019): 337–360, https://onlinelibrary .wiley.com/doi/abs/10.1111/socf.12500.

9. Nico S. Rizzo, Karen Jaceldo-Siegl, Joan Sabate, and Gary E. Fraser, "Nutrient Profiles of Vegetarian and Nonvegetarian Dietary Patterns," *Journal of the Academy of Nutrition and Dietetics* 113, no. 12 (2013): 1610–19, https://pubmed .ncbi.nlm.nih.gov/23988511/.

10. Nick Fiddes, *Meat: A Natural Symbol* (Oxfordshire, UK: Routledge, 1992), 42.

11. Oldways, "Plant-Based Heritage," September 21, 2022, https://oldwayspt .org/blog/plant-based-heritage.

12. Elizabeth Cherry, *Culture and Activism: Animal Rights in France and the United States* (Oxfordshire, UK: Routledge, 2010), 469.

13. Nathaniel Popper, "This Animal Activist Used to Get in Your Face. Now He's Going After Your Palate," *New York Times*, March 12, 2019, https://www.nytimes.com/2019/03/12/technology/bruce-friedrich-animal-activist.html.

14. Jonathan A. Foley, "5 Steps to Feed the World and Sustain the Planet," *Scientific American*, June 1, 2015, https://www.scientificamerican.com/article/5-steps-to-feed-the-world-and-sustain-the-planet

CHAPTER THREE: MAKING "MEAT"

1. Connecticut College, "The Vegan Entrepreneur," April 2, 2015, https://conncoll.edu/academics/vegan-entrepreneur/.

2. Marc Gunther, "The Bill Gates-Backed Company That's Reinventing Meat," *Fortune*, October 3, 2013, https://fortune.com/2013/10/03/the-bill-gates-backed-company-thats-reinventing-meat/.

3. "Here Are Beyond Meat's Biggest—and Happiest—Investors," *CBInsights*, June 6, 2019, https://cbinsights.com/research/beyond-meat-ipo-investor-analysis/.

4. Bill Gates, "Future of Food," *Gates Notes*, March 18, 2013, https://gatesnotes.com/future-of-food.

5. William Shurtleff and Akiko Aoyagi, "History of Tofu—Page 1," SoyInfo Center, 2004, https://soyinfocenter.com/HSS/tofu1.php.

6. Brian Cooley, "Beyond Burgers Now Ship to Your Door," *CNET*, June 11, 2019, https://cnet.com/health/nutrition/new-beyond-burger-unveiled-that-tastes-looks-eerily-more-like-beef/.

7. Gosia Wozniacka, "Plant-Based Diets and Regenerative Ag Have Sparked a Pea and Lentil Renaissance," *Civil Eats*, February 18, 2020, https://civileats.com/2020/02/18/plant-based-diets-and-regenerative-ag-have-sparked-a-pea-and-lentil-renaissance/.

8. Rebecca Schouten, "Beyond Meat Unveils Two New Beyond Burger Iterations," *Food Business News*, November 16, 2020, https://foodbusinessnews.net/articles/17304-beyond-meat-unveils-two-new-beyond-burger-iterations.

9. Niamh Michail, "What Are the Best Colour Options for Plant-Based Meats?" *Food Navigator USA*, May 16, 2018, https://foodnavigator.com/Article/2018/05/16/What-are-the-best-colour-options-for-plant-based-meats.

10. Marion Nestle, "Plant-Based Meat: The Cosmetic Color Problem," *Food Politics*, May 22, 2018, https://foodpolitics.com/tag/meat-substitutes/page/3/.

11. Larissa G. Baraldi, Euridice Martinez Steele, Daniela Silva Canella, and Carlos Augusto Monteiro, "Consumption of Ultra-Processed Foods and Associated Sociodemographic Factors in the USA Between 2007 and 2012: Evidence from a Nationally Representative Cross-Sectional Study," *BMJ Open* 8, no. 3 (2018): e020574, https://pubmed.ncbi.nlm.nih.gov/29525772/.

12. Gwen Pearson, "You Know What Makes Great Food Coloring? Bugs," *WIRED*, September 9, 2015, https://wired.com/2015/09/cochineal-bug-feature/.

13. Good Food Institute, "2021 U.S. Retail Market Insights for the Plant-Based Industry," 2021, https://gfi.org/marketresearch/.

14. Miyoko Schinner, LinkedIn, April 2022, https://linkedin.com/posts/miyoko-schinner-6a47204_im-sorry-if-i-disappoint-but-my-company-activity-6921629516226334720-P6Zn.

CHAPTER FOUR: MEAT WITHOUT MISERY

1. John Evans and Drew Cherry, "Two Years Ago, Cell-Based Salmon Cost $200,000 per Pound to Manufacture. Today, It's a Fraction of That Cost," *IntraFish*, June 7, 2022, https://intrafish.com/technology/two-years-ago-cell-based-salmon-cost-200-000-per-pound-to-manufacture-today-its-a-fraction-of-that-cost-/2-1-1231452.

2. Our World in Data, "Global Fish Production," 2022, https://ourworldindata.org/fish-and-overfishing.

3. Food and Agriculture Organization of the United Nations, "FAO Members Endorse Declaration for Sustainable Fisheries and Aquaculture," *Globefish*, December 2, 2021, https://fao.org/in-action/globefish/news-events/details-news/en/c/1374953/.

4. Our World in Data, "Seafood Production: Wild Fish Catch vs. Aquaculture, World," June 6, 2022, https://ourworldindata.org/grapher/capture-fisheries -vs-aquaculture.

5. Food and Agriculture Organization of the United Nations, "The State of World Fisheries and Aquaculture," August 19, 2022, https://www.fao.org/documents /card/en?details=cc0461en.

6. Sarah Gibbens, "Less than 3 Percent of the Ocean is 'Highly Protected,'" *National Geographic*, September 25, 2019, https://nationalgeographic.com /environment/article/paper-parks-undermine-marine-protected-areas.

7. Ling-Feng Zeng et al., "An Exploration of the Role of a Fish-Oriented Diet in Cognitive Decline: A Systematic Review of the Literature," *Oncotarget* 8, no. 24 (2017): 39877, https://www.ncbi.nlm.nih.gov/pmc/articles/PMC5503660/.

8. Winston Churchill, "Fifty Years Hence," *Strand*, December 1931, https://www .nationalchurchillmuseum.org/fifty-years-hence.html.

9. Wendy Wolfson, "Lab-Grown Steaks Nearing the Menu," *New Scientist*, December 30, 2022, https://newscientist.com/article/dn3208-lab-grown-steaks -nearing-the-menu/.

10. Michael Specter, "Test-Tube Burgers," *New Yorker*, May 16, 2011, https://www .newyorker.com/magazine/2011/05/23/test-tube-burgers.

11. New Harvest, "How the New Harvest Community Coined the Term Cellular Agriculture," March 27, 2021, https://new-harvest.org/community-coined -cellular-agriculture/.

12. Isha Datar and Mirko Betti, "Possibilities for an In-Vitro Meat Production System," *Innovative Food Science and Emerging Technologies* 11, no. 1 (2010): 13–22, https://doi.org/10.1016/j.ifset.2009.10.007.

13. Neil Stephens, Alexandra E. Sexton, and Clemens Driessen, "Making Sense of Making Meat: Key Moments in the First 20 Years of Tissue Engineering Muscle to Make Food," *Frontiers in Sustainable Food Systems* 3, no. 45 (2019): 16, https://www.frontiersin.org/articles/10.3389/fsufs.2019.00045/full.

14. Sam Harris, "Meat without Misery: A Conversation with Uma Valeti," *Making Sense* podcast, February 19, 2016, https://samharris.org/podcasts/making-sense-episodes/meat-without-murder.

15. Jeff Bercovici, "Why This Cardiologist Is Betting That His Lab-Grown Meat Startup Can Solve the Global Food Crisis," *Inc.*, October 24, 2017, https://inc.com/magazine/201711/jeff-bercovici/memphis-meats-lab-grown-meat-startup.html.

16. Ezra Klein, "Let's Launch a Moonshot for Meatless Meat," *New York Times*, April 24, 2021, https://nytimes.com/2021/04/24/opinion/climate-change-meatless-meat.html.

17. David Humbird, "Scale-Up Economics for Cultured Meat," *Biotechnology and Bioengineering* 118, no. 8 (June 7, 2021): 3239–50, https://onlinelibrary.wiley.com/doi/10.1002/bit.27848.

18. Joe Fassler, "Lab-Grown Meat Is Supposed to Be Inevitable. The Science Tells a Different Story," *Counter*, September 22, 2021, https://thecounter.org/lab-grown-cultivated-meat-cost-at-scale/.

19. Erin McCormick, "Eat Just Is Racing to Put 'No-Kill Meat' on Your Plate. Is It Too Good to Be True?" *Guardian*, June 16, 2021, https://theguardian.com/food/2021/jun/16/eat-just-no-kill-meat-chicken-josh-tetrick.

20. Nicola Jones, "Food: A Taste of Things to Come?" *Nature* 468 (2010): 752–53, https://nature.com/articles/468752a.

21. Joseph Mohorčich and Jacy Reese, "Cell-Cultured Meat: Lessons from GMO Adoption and Resistance," *Appetite* 143, no. 1 (2019), https://sciencedirect.com/science/article/abs/pii/S0195666319304829.

22. U.S. Food and Drug Administration, "Human Food Made with Cultured Animal Cells Inventory," November 14, 2022, https://cfsanappsexternal.fda.gov/scripts/fdcc/?set=AnimalCellCultureFoods&id=002.

23. H. L. Tuomisto and M. J. de Mattos, "Environmental Impacts of Cultured Meat Production," *Environmental Science and Technology* 45, no. 14 (2011): 6117–6123, https://pubs.acs.org/doi/10.1021/es200130u.

24. H. L. Tuomisto, Scott J. Allan, and Marianne J. Ellis, "Prospective Life Cycle Assessment of a Bioprocess Design for Cultured Meat Production in Hollow Fiber Bioreactors," *Science of the Total Environment* 851, no. 10 (2022): 1–11, https://sciencedirect.com/science/article/pii/S0048969722051506.

25. Sergiy Smetana, Alexander Mathys, Achim Knoch, and Volker Heinz, "Meat Alternatives: Life Cycle Assessment of Most Known Meat Substitutes," *International Journal of Life Cycle Assessment* 20, no. 9 (2015): 1254–67, https://link .springer.com/article/10.1007/s11367-015-0931-6.

26. Adele Peters, "What's the Carbon Footprint of Lab-Grown Meat?" *Fast Company*, March 9, 2021, https://fastcompany.com/90612190/whats-the -carbon-footprint-of-lab-grown-meat.

27. National Cattlemen's Beef Association, "NCBA Applauds U.S. Senate Introduction of Real MEAT Act," 2019, https://ncba.org/ncba-news/news-releases /news/details/25948/ncba-applauds-us-senate-introduction-of-real-meat-act.

28. Hannah Ritchie, "How Do We Reduce Antibiotic Resistance from Livestock?" Our World in Data, 2020, https://ourworldindata.org/grapher/antibiotic -usage-in-livestock.

29. Stephanie J. Salyer, Rachel Silver, Kerri Simone, and Casey B. Behravesh, "Prioritizing Zoonoses for Global Health Capacity Building: Themes from One Health Zoonotic Disease Workshops in 7 Countries, 2014–2016," *Emerging Infectious Diseases* 23, no. 13 (2017): S55–64, https://pubmed.ncbi.nlm.nih.gov/29155664/.

30. Brave Robot, "The Process Behind the Magic," 2022, https://braverobot.co /pages/process.

CHAPTER FIVE: THE VEGAN MAFIA

1. Good Food Institute, "Record $3.1 Billion Invested in Alt Proteins in 2020 Signals Growing Market Momentum for Sustainable Protein," March 18, 2021, https://gfi.org/blog/2020-state-of-the-industry-highlights/.

2. Good Food Institute, *2020 State of the Industry Report: Plant-Based Meat, Eggs, and Dairy*, https://gfi.org/plant-based/.

3. Good Food Institute, *2020 State of the Industry Report: Cultivated Meat*, https://gfi.org/cultivated/.

4. Good Food Institute, *2020 State of the Industry Report: Fermentation: Meat, Seafood, Eggs, and Dairy*, https://gfi.org/fermentation/.

5. Howard B. Lewis, "Proteins in Nutrition," *JAMA*, September 18, 1948, https://jamanetwork.com/journals/jama/article-abstract/301397.

6. USDA, 2014, "What We Eat in America," *NHANES*, 2011–2012, Washington, D.C., https://ars.usda.gov/northeast-area/beltsville-md-bhnrc/beltsville-human-nutrition-research-center/food-surveys-research-group/docs/wweianhanes-overview/.

7. Michael Huesemann and Joyce Huesemann, *Techno-Fix: Why Technology Won't Save Us or the Environment* (New York: New Society Publishers, 2011), 3.

8. Warren Belasco, *Meals to Come: A History of the Future of Food* (Berkeley: University of California Press, 2006), 55.

9. Marion Nestle, *Food Politics: How the Food Industry Influences Nutrition and Health* (Berkeley: University of California Press, 2013), 4.

10. Matt McGrath, "Climate Change: IPCC Report Is 'Code Red for Humanity,'" *BBC News*, August 9, 2021, https://bbc.com/news/science-environment-58130705.

11. Jessica L. Johnston, Jessica C. Fanzo, and Bruce Cogill, "Understanding Sustainable Diets: A Descriptive Analysis of the Determinants and Processes That Influence Diets and Their Impact on Health, Food Security, and Environmental Sustainability," *Advances in Nutrition* 5, no. 4 (2014): 418–29, https://www.ncbi.nlm.nih.gov/pmc/articles/PMC4085190/.

CHAPTER SIX: LET THEM EAT GRASS-FED BEEF

1. Edible Education, "The What, Why, and How of Regenerative Agriculture," February 5, 2020, https://edibleschoolyard.org/ee101-2020.

2. Klaus Weber, Kathryn L. Heinze, and Michaela DeSoucey, "Forage for Thought: Mobilizing Codes in the Movement for Grass-Fed Meat and Dairy

Products," *Administrative Science Quarterly* 53, no. 3 (2008): 528–67, https:// journals.sagepub.com/doi/10.2189/asqu.53.3.529.

3. Rodale Institute, "Regenerative Organic Agriculture," 2023, https://rodalein stitute.org/why-organic/organic-basics/regenerative-organic-agriculture/.

4. David D. Briske, Brandon T. Bestelmeyer, Joel R. Brown, Samuel D. Fuhlendorf, and H. Wayne Polley, "The Savory Method Can Not Green Deserts or Reverse Climate Change: A Response to the Allan Savory TED Video," *Rangelands* 35, no. 5 (2013): 72–74, https://repository.arizona.edu/handle /10150/639967.

5. Tara Garnett, Cécile Godde, Adrian Muller, Elin Röös, Pete Smith, Imke de Boer, Erasmus zu Ermgassen, Mario Herrero, Corina van Middelaar, Christian Schader, and Hannah van Zanten, "Grazed and Confused?" *FCRN*, October 1, 2017, https://tabledebates.org/publication/grazed-and-confused.

6. Matthew N. Hayek and Rachael D. Garrett, "Nationwide Shift to Grass-Fed Beef Requires Larger Cattle Population," *Environmental Research Letters* 13 (2018): 1–8, https://iopscience.iop.org/article/10.1088/1748-9326/aad401/meta.

7. Hannah Ritchie, "How Much of the World's Land Would We Need in Order to Feed the Global Population with the Average Diet of a Given Country?" Our World in Data, October 3, 2017, https://ourworldindata.org/agricultural -land-by-global-diets.

8. H. Charles J. Godfray, Paul Aveyard, Tara Garnett, Jim H. Hall, Timothy J. Key, Jamie Lorimer, Ray T. Pierrehumbert, Peter Scarborough, Marco Springmann, and Susan A. Jebb, "Meat Consumption, Health, and the Environment," *Science* 361, no. 6399 (2018), https://science.org/doi/10.1126/science.aam5324.

9. Matthew N. Hayek, Helen Harwatt, William J. Ripple, and Nathaniel D. Mueller, "The Carbon Opportunity Cost of Animal-Sourced Food Production on Land," *Nature Sustainability* 4 (2021): 21–24, https://nature.com/articles /s41893-020-00603-4.

10. Bernardo B. N. Strassburg et al., "Global Priority Areas for Ecosystem Restoration," *Nature* 586 (2020): 724–29, https://nature.com/articles/s41586-020 -2784-9#auth-Carlos_Leandro-Cordeiro.

11. Michael A. Clark, Nina G. Domingo, Kimberly Colgan, Sumil K. Thakrar, David Tilman, John Lynch, Inês L. Azevedo, and Jason D. Hill, "Global Food System Emissions Could Preclude Achieving the 1.5° and 2°C Climate Change Targets," *Science* 370, no. 6517 (2020), https://science.org/doi/10.1126/science.aba7357.

12. Oren Shelef, Peter J. Weidberg, and Frederick D. Provenza, "The Value of Native Plants and Local Production in an Era of Global Agriculture," *Frontiers in Plant Science* (2017), https://ncbi.nlm.nih.gov/pmc/articles/PMC5723411/.

13. Keith Paustian, Eric Larson, Jeffrey Kent, Ernie Marx, and Amy Swan, "Soil C Sequestration as a Biological Negative Emission Strategy," *Frontiers in Climate* 1 (2019), https://frontiersin.org/articles/10.3389/fclim.2019.00008/full.

14. Michael Pollan, "Unhappy Meals," *New York Times Magazine*, January 28, 2007, https://nytimes.com/2007/01/28/magazine/28nutritionism.t.html.

15. Joshua Specht, *Red Meat Republic: A Hoof-to-Table History of How Beef Changed America* (Princeton, NJ: Princeton University Press, 2019).

16. Jan Dutkiewicz and Gabriel N. Rosenberg, "The Myth of Regenerative Ranching," *New Republic*, September 23, 2021, https://newrepublic.com/article/163735/myth-regenerative-ranching.

17. Erica Gies, "Unique Elk in California May be Killed Under Controversial Plan," *National Geographic*, September 30, 2020, https://nationalgeographic.com/animals/article/tule-elk-culled-under-point-reyes-proposal.

CHAPTER SEVEN: FROM THE GROUND UP

1. Karl Blankenship, "Chesapeake Bay Cleanup Faces Difficult Trade-offs with Agriculture," *Bay Journal*, May 1, 2023, https://www.bayjournal.com/news/policy/chesapeake-bay-cleanup-faces-difficult-trade-offs-with-agriculture/article_896365bc-e43b-11ed-beac-b396d2795ed7.html

2. Kristine Wong, "Will This Maryland Bill Get Big Chicken to Clean Up Its Act?" *Civil Eats*, January 26, 2016, https://civileats.com/2016/01/26/will-this-maryland-bill-get-big-chicken-to-clean-up-its-act-chesapeake-bay/.

3. Julie E. Kurtz, Peter B. Woodbury, Zia U. Ahmed, and Christian J. Peters, "Mapping U.S. Food System Localization Potential: The Impact of Diet on Foodsheds," *Environmental Science & Technology* 54, no. 19 (2020): 12434-12446, https://pubs.acs.org/doi/10.1021/acs.est.9b07582.

4. Eliot Coleman, *The New Organic Grower, 3rd Edition: A Master's Manual of Tools and Techniques for the Home and Market Gardener* (White River Junction, VT: Chelsea Green Publishing, 2018)

CHAPTER EIGHT: YOU ARE WHAT YOU EAT

1. E. Melanie Dupuis, *Nature's Perfect Food* (New York: NYU Press, 2002)

2. Ethan Varian, "It's Called 'Plant-Based,' Look It Up," *New York Times*, December 28, 2019, https://nytimes.com/2019/12/28/style/plant-based-diet.html.

3. T. Colin Campbell, "History of the Term 'Whole Food, Plant-Based,'" T. Colin Campbell Center for Nutrition Studies, November 29, 2016 (updated January 4, 2019), https://nutritionstudies.org/history-of-the-term-whole-food -plant-based/.

4. T. Colin Campbell and Junshi Chen, "Diet and Chronic Degenerative Diseases: Perspectives from China," *American Journal of Clinical Nutrition* 59, no. 5 (1994): 1153S–61S, https://pubmed.ncbi.nlm.nih.gov/8172116/.

5. T. Colin Campbell, Banoo Parpia, and Junshi Chen, "Diet, Lifestyle, and the Etiology of Coronary Artery Disease: The Cornell China Study," *American Journal of Cardiology* 82, no. 10 (1998): 18–21, https://pubmed.ncbi.nlm.nih.gov /9860369/.

6. Jane E. Brody, "Huge Study of Diet Indicts Fat and Meat," *New York Times*, May 8, 1990, https://nytimes.com/1990/05/08/science/huge-study-of-diet -indicts-fat-and-meat.html.

7. Jiaqi Huang et al., "Association Between Plant and Animal Protein Intake and Overall and Cause-Specific Mortality," *JAMA Internal Medicine* 180, no. 9 (2020): 1173–84, https://jamanetwork.com/journals/jamainternalmedicine /fullarticle/2768358.

8. Mingyang Song et al., "Association of Animal and Plant Protein Intake with All-Cause and Cause-Specific Mortality," *JAMA Internal Medicine* 176, no. 10 (2016): 1453–63, https://jamanetwork.com/journals/jamainternalmedicine/fullarticle/2540540.

9. Christopher D. Gardner, Jennifer C. Hartle, Rachael D. Garrett, Lisa C. Offringa, and Arlin S. Wasserman, "Maximizing the Intersection of Human Health and the Environment with Regard to the Amount and Type of Protein Produced and Consumed in the United States," *Nutrition Reviews* 1, no. 77 (2019): 197–215, https://pubmed.ncbi.nlm.nih.gov/30726996/.

10. Gwenyth K. Davey, Elizabeth A. Spencer, Paul N. Appleby, Naomi E. Allen, Katherine H. Knox, and Timothy J. Key, "EPIC–Oxford: Lifestyle Character-istics and Nutrient Intakes in a Cohort of 33 883 Meat-Eaters and 31 546 Non Meat-Eaters in the UK," *Public Health Nutrition* 6, no. 3 (2003): 259–68, https://pubmed.ncbi.nlm.nih.gov/12740075/.

11. Sara B. Seidelmann et al., "Dietary Carbohydrate Intake and Mortality: A Prospective Cohort Study and Meta-Analysis," *Lancet Public Health* 3(9) (2018): e419–28, https://www.thelancet.com/journals/lanpub/article/PIIS2468-2667(18)30135-X.

12. Brody, "Huge Study of Diet."

13. Caldwell Esselstyn, "A Plant-Based Diet and Coronary Artery Disease: A Mandate for Effective Therapy," *Journal of Geriatric Cardiology* 14, no. 5 (2017): 317–20, https://pubmed.ncbi.nlm.nih.gov/28630609/.

14. Cristina-Mihaela Lăcătuşu, Elena-Daniela Grigorescu, Mariana Floria, Alina Onofriescu, Bogdan-Mircea Mihai, "The Mediterranean Diet: From an Environment-Driven Food Culture to an Emerging Medical Prescription," *International Journal of Environmental Research and Public Health* 16, no. 6 (2019): 942, https://www.ncbi.nlm.nih.gov/pmc/articles/PMC6466433/.

15. Neal D. Barnard et al., "A Mediterranean Diet and Low-Fat Vegan Diet to Improve Body Weight and Cardiometabolic Risk Factors: A Randomized,

Cross-Over Trial," *Journal of the American College of Nutrition* (2020): 1–13, https://pubmed.ncbi.nlm.nih.gov/33544066/.

16. J. M. Pettifor, "Calcium and Vitamin D Metabolism in Children in Developing Countries," *Annals of Nutrition and Metabolism* 64, Suppl. 2 (2014): 15–22, https://pubmed.ncbi.nlm.nih.gov/25341870/.

17. Walter C. Willett and David S. Ludwig, 2020. "Milk and Health," *New England Journal of Medicine* 382(7): 644–54, https://www.nejm.org/doi/full/10.1056 /NEJMra1903547.

18. Renata Micha, Jose L. Peñalvo, Frederick Cudhea, Fumiaki Imamura, Colin D. Rehm, and Dariush Mozaffarian, "Association Between Dietary Factors and Mortality from Heart Disease, Stroke, and Type 2 Diabetes in the United States," *JAMA* 317, no. 9 (2017): 912–24, https://pubmed.ncbi.nlm.nih.gov /28267855/.

19. Ashkan Afshin et al., "Health Effects of Dietary Risks in 195 Countries, 1990–2017: A Systematic Analysis for the Global Burden of Disease Study 2017," *Lancet* 393, no. 10184 (2019): 1958–72, https://sciencedirect.com/science /article/pii/S0140673619300418.

20. Institute for Health Metrics and Evaluation, "Global Burden of Disease (GBD)," 2019, https://healthdata.org/research-analysis/gbd.

21. Nathaniel P. Morris, "The Neglect of Nutrition in Medical Education: A First-hand Look," *JAMA Internal Medicine* 174, no. 6 (2014): 841–42, https://jama network.com/journals/jamainternalmedicine/article-abstract/1860501.

22. David Katz, "Lifestyle Is the Medicine, Culture Is the Spoon: The Covariance of Proposition and Preposition," *American Journal of Lifestyle Medicine* 8 (2014): 301–305, https://doi:10.1177/1559827614527720.

23. Dean Ornish and Anne Ornish, *Undo It!* (New York: Random House, 2019), 241.

24. Dean Ornish, L. W. Scherwitz, R. S. Doody, D. Kesten, S. M. McLanahan, S. E. Brown, E. DePuey, R. Sonnemaker, C. Haynes, J. Lester, G. K. McAllister,

R. J. Hall, J. A. Burdine, and A. M. Gotto, Jr., "Effects of Stress Management Training and Dietary Changes in Treating Ischemic Heart Disease," *JAMA* 248, no. 1 (1983): 54–59, https://jamanetwork.com/journals/jama/article-abs tract/381576.

25. Dean Ornish, S. E. Brown, L. W. Scherwitz, J. H. Billings, W. T. Armstrong, T. A. Ports, S. M. McLanahan, R. L. Kirkeeide, R. J. Brand, and K. L. Gould, "Can Lifestyle Changes Reverse Coronary Heart Disease? The Lifestyle Heart Trial," *Lancet* 336, no. 8708 (1990): 129–33, https://pubmed.ncbi.nlm.nih.gov /1973470/.

26. Dean Ornish, M. J. M. Magbanua, G. Weidner, V. Weinberg, C. Kemp, C. Green, M. D. Marlin, J. Simko, K. Shinohara, C. M. Haqq, and P. R. Carroll, "Changes in Prostate Gene Expression in Men Undergoing an Intensive Nutrition and Lifestyle Intervention," *Proceedings of the National Academy of Sciences U.S.A.* 105, no. 24 (2008): 8369–74, https://www.ncbi.nlm.nih.gov /pmc/articles/PMC2430265/.

27. Christopher D. Gardner, John F. Trepanowski, Liana C. Del Gobbo, Michelle E. Hauser, Joseph Rigdon, John P. A. Ioannidis, Manisha Desai, and Abby C. King, "Effect of Low-Fat vs Low-Carbohydrate Diet on 12-Month Weight Loss in Overweight Adults and the Association with Genotype Pattern or Insulin Secretion: The DIETFITS Randomized Clinical Trial," *JAMA* 319, no. 7 (2018): 667–79, https://pubmed.ncbi.nlm.nih.gov/29466592/.

28. Walter C. Willett, "Balancing Lifestyle and Genomics Research for Disease Prevention," *Science* 296, no. 5568 (2002): 695–98, https://pubmed.ncbi.nlm .nih.gov/11976443/.

29. Elizabeth Blackburn and Elissa Epel, *The Telomere Effect: A Revolutionary Approach to Living Younger, Healthier, Longer* (New York: Grand Central, 2017).

30. Dean Ornish, J. Lin, J. M. Chan, E. Epel, C. Jemp, G. Weidner, R. Marlin, S. J. Frenda, M. J. M. Magbanua, J. Daubenmier, I. Estay, N. K. Hills, N. Chainani-Wu, P. T. Carroll, and E. H. Blackburn, "Effect of Comprehensive Lifestyle Changes on Telomerase Activity and Telomere Length in Men with Biopsy-Proven Low-Risk Prostate Cancer: 5-Year Follow-Up of a Descriptive Pilot

Study," *Lancet Oncology* 14, no. 11 (2013): 1112–20, https://pubmed.ncbi.nlm.nih .gov/24051140/.

31. CMS.gov, "Decision Memo for Intensive Cardiac Rehabilitation (ICR) Program: Dr. Dean Ornish's Program for Reversing Heart Disease," August 12, 2010, https://www.cms.gov/medicare-coverage-database/view/ncacal-decision -memo.aspx?proposed=N&NCAId=240&NcaName=Intensive+Cardiac +Rehabilitation+%28ICR%29+Program+-+Dr.+Ornish.

32. Dean Ornish, "The Myth of High-Protein Diets," *New York Times*, March 23, 2015, https://www.nytimes.com/2015/03/23/opinion/the-myth-of-high-protein -diets.html.

33. Pan An, Qi Sun, Adam M. Bernstein, Matthias B. Schulze, JoAnn E. Manson, Meir J. Stampfer, Walter C. Willett, and Frank B. Hu, "Red Meat Consump- tion and Mortality: Results from 2 Prospective Cohort Studies," *Archives of Internal Medicine* 9, no. 172 (2012): 555–63, https://pubmed.ncbi.nlm.nih.gov /22412075/.

34. Ornish and Ornish, *Undo It!*, 66.

35. Craig J. Winston and Ann Reed Mangels, "Position of the American Dietetic Association: Vegetarian Diets," *Journal of the American Dietetic Association* 109, no. 7 (2009): 1266–82, https://pubmed.ncbi.nlm.nih.gov/19562864/.

36. Emanuele Di Angelantonio et al, "Body-Mass Index and All-Cause Mortality: Individual-Participant-Data Meta-Analysis of 239 Prospective Studies in Four Continents," *Lancet* 388, no. 10046 (2016), 776–86, https://www.thelancet.com /journals/lancet/article/PIIS0140-67361630175-1.

37. Ornish and Ornish, *Undo It!*, 33.

38. Alzheimer's Association, "Alzheimer's Disease Facts and Figures Annual Report," 2023, https://www.alz.org/media/Documents/alzheimers-facts-and -figures.pdf .

39. J. Verheijen and K. Sleegers, "Understanding Alzheimer Disease at the Inter- face Between Genetics and Transcriptomics," *Trends in Genetics* 34, no. 6 (2018), 434–47, https://pubmed.ncbi.nlm.nih.gov/29573818/.

40. Dean Sherzai and Ayesha Sherzai, *The Alzheimer's Solution: A Revolutionary Guide to How You Can Prevent and Reverse Memory Loss* (London: Simon and Schuster, 2017).

41. Clare Martha Morris, Denis A. Evans, Julia L Bienias, Christine C. Tangney, David A. Bennett, Neelum Aggarwal, Julie Schneider, and Robert S. Wilson, "Dietary Fats and the Risk of Incident Alzheimer's Disease," *Arch Neurol* 60, no. 2 (2003): 194–200, https://pubmed.ncbi.nlm.nih.gov/12580703/.

42. A. Solomon, M. Kivipelto, B. Wolozin, J. Zhou, and R. A. Whitmer, "Midlife Serum Cholesterol and Increased Risk of Alzheimer's and Vascular Dementia Three Decades Later," *Dementia and Geriatric Cognitive Disorders* 28, no. 1 (2009): 75–80, https://pubmed.ncbi.nlm.nih.gov/19648749/.

43. Jing Wu et al., "Dietary Pattern in Midlife and Cognitive Impairment in Late Life: A Prospective Study in Chinese Adults," *American Journal of Clinical Nutrition* 110, no. 4 (2019): 912–20, https://pubmed.ncbi.nlm.nih.gov/31374567/.

44. Klodian Dhana, Denis A. Evans, Kumar B. Rajan, David A. Bennett, and Martha C. Morris, "Healthy Lifestyle and the Risk of Alzheimer Dementia: Findings from 2 Longitudinal Studies," *Neurology* 95, no. 4 (2020): e374–83, https://pubmed.ncbi.nlm.nih.gov/32554763/.

CHAPTER NINE: CULT TO COOL

1. Pete Wells, "The Garden, Both Muse and Oracle at L'Arpège," *New York Times*, May 6, 2014, https://nytimes.com/2014/05/07/dining/the-garden-both-muse -and-oracle-at-larpege.html.

2. Harriet Agnew, "Take a Look Around Parisian Super-Chef Alain Passard's Medieval Château," *Financial Times*, October 4, 2019, https://ft.com/content /98c46142-da02-11e9-8f9b-77216ebe1f17.

3. "Alain Passard: In the Kitchen (and Garden) with the Michelin-Starred Chef," *FT Life*, Meaningful Pursuits, November 12, 2019, https://youtube.com /watch?v=xrwfIj9gfy4&t=206s.

4. Although the original article was deleted, the same statement can be found in the following report: Ministère de la santé, de la famille, et des personnes

handicapées, "La santé vient en mangeant: Le guide alimentaire pour tous,"
2002, https://solidarites-sante.gouv.fr/IMG/pdf/guide_alimentairetous.pdf.

5. Micaela DeSoucey, "Gastronationalism: Food Traditions and Authenticity
Politics in the European Union." *American Sociological Review* 75, no. 3 (2010):
432–55, https://doi.org/10.1177/0003122410372226.

6. France Télévisions, "Faut-il arrêter de manger de la viande?" *C à vous*, June 28,
2018, youtube.com/watch?v=ugskBKfu7gY&t=1055s.

7. Brett Anderson and Jenny Gross, "The New Menu at Eleven Madison Park
Will Be Meatless," *New York Times*, May 3, 2021, nytimes.com/2021/05/03
/dining/eleven-madison-park-vegan-menu.html.

8. Ibid.

CHAPTER TEN: SOUL FOOD

1. Dalia Colón and Kimberly Vlach, "Comedian, Activist Dick Gregory Talks
Health," *TheHealthyState*, 2011, https://youtube.com/watch?v=vcwza6YBF3M.

2. Justin McCarthy and Scott DeKoster, "Nearly One in Four in U.S. Have Cut
Back on Eating Meat," Gallup, January 27, 2020, https://news.gallup.com/poll
/282779/nearly-one-four-cut-back-eating-meat.aspx.

3. Jonathan Kauffman, *Hippie Food: How Back-to-the-Landers, Longhairs, and
Revolutionaries Changed the Way We Eat* (New York: HarperCollins, 2019), 13.

4. Amirah Mercer, "A Homecoming," *Eater*, January 14, 2021, https://www.eater
.com/22229322/black-veganism-history-black-panthers-dick-gregory-nation
-of-islam-alvenia-fulton.

5. Angela Davis, "Angela Davis on Veganism as Part of a Revolutionary Perspective," *Films for Action*, 2012, https://www.filmsforaction.org/watch/angela
-davis-on-veganism-as-part-of-a-revolutionary-perspective/.

6. Monica Webb Hooper, Vanessa Marshall, and Eliseo J. Pérez-Stable,
"COVID-19 Health Disparities and Adverse Social Determinants of Health,"
Behav Med 48, no. 2 (2022): 133–40, https://pubmed.ncbi.nlm.nih.gov/35
318895/.

7. Frederick Douglass Opie, *Hog and Hominy: Soul Food from Africa to America* (New York: Columbia University Press, 2008), 132.

8. Jessica B. Harris, *High on the Hog: A Culinary Journey from Africa to America* (New York: Bloomsbury, 2011), 15.

9. Nir Avieli, and Franc Markowitz, "Slavery Food, Soul Food, Salvation Food: Veganism and Identity in the African Hebrew Israelite Community," *African and Black Diaspora: An International Journal* 11, no. 2 (2018): 205–20, https://www.tandfonline.com/doi/abs/10.1080/17528631.2017.1394612.

10. Ronit Vered, "The Hebrew Israelite's Secret to Eternal Life," *Haaretz*, 2016. https://www.haaretz.com/food/2016-04-09/ty-article-magazine/.premium/the -hebrew-israelites-secret-to-eternal-life/0000017f-f446-d47e-a37f-fd7ed9010000.

11. Bryant Terry, *Vegan Soul Kitchen* (New York: Hachette, 2009), 30.

12. Punam Ohri-Vachaspati, Zeynep Isgor, Leah Rimkus, Lisa M. Powell, Dianne C. Barket, and Frank J. Chaloupka, "Child-Directed Marketing Inside and on the Exterior of Fast-Food Restaurants," *AJPM* 48, no. 1 (2014): 22–30. https://www.ajpmonline.org/article/S0749-3797(14)00478-4/fulltext#%20.

13. Pierre Bourdieu, *Distinction: A Social Critique of the Judgment of Taste* (Cambridge, MA: Harvard University Press, 1987). Translated by Richard Nice.

14. Emily H. Kennedy, Shyon Baumann, and Josée Johnston, "Eating for Taste and Eating for Change: Ethical Consumption as a High-Status Practice," *Social Forces* 98, no. 1 (2019): 381–402, https://academic.oup.com/sf/article-abstract /98/1/381/5239860.

15. Daniel L. Rosenfeld, "The Psychology of Vegetarianism: Recent Advances and Future Directions," *Appetite* 131, no. 1 (2018): 125–38, https://www.sciencedirect .com/science/article/abs/pii/S0195666318309309..

16. McCarthy and DeKoster, "Nearly One in Four in U.S."

17. Michael W. Twitty, *The Cooking Gene: A Journey Through African American Culinary History in the Old South* (New York: Amistad, 2017), 269.

18. Ron Finely, "A Guerrilla Gardener in South Central LA," TED talk, February 2013, https://ted.com/talks/ron_finley_a_guerrilla_gardener_in _south_central_la?language=en#t-618158.

CHAPTER ELEVEN: THE PAST OF FOOD

1. Hannah Ritchie, "Soy," Our World in Data, June 2021, https://ourworldindata .org/soy.

2. World Wildlife Fund, "The Growth of Soy: Impacts and Solutions," *WWF International*, 2014, https://wwf.panda.org/wwf_news/?214091/The-Growth-of -Soy-Impacts-and-Solutions.

3. Francis Moore Lappé, *Diet for a Small Planet* (New York: Ballantine Books, 1991), 13.

4. Kevin D. Hall et al., "Effect of a Plant-Based, Low-Fat Diet Versus an Animal-Based, Ketogenic Diet on Ad Libitum Energy Intake," *Nature Medicine* 27 (2021): 344–53, https://pubmed.ncbi.nlm.nih.gov/33479499/.

5. Thomas L. Robertson et al., "Epidemiologic Studies of Coronary Heart Disease and Stroke in Japanese Men Living in Japan, Hawaii, and California: Incidence of Myocardial Infarction and Death from Coronary Heart Disease," *American Journal of Cardiology* 39, no. 2 (1977): 239–43, https://pubmed.ncbi.nlm .nih.gov/835482/.

6. Rachel Ann Delicano, Ulf Hammar, Agneta Egenvall, Carri Westgarth, Mwenya Mubanga, Liisa Byberg, Tove Fall, and Beatrice Kennedy, "The Shared Risk of Diabetes Between Dog and Cat Owners and Their Pets: Register Based Cohort Study," *BMJ* 371 (2020): 4337, https://www.bmj.com/content/371/bmj.m4337.

7. John McDougall and Mary McDougall, *The Starch Solution: Eat the Foods You Love, Regain Your Health, and Lose the Weight for Good!* (New York: Rodale Books, 2012).

8. Max Roser, Esteban Ortiz-Ospina, and Hannah Ritchie, "Life Expectancy," Our World in Data, 2019, https://ourworldindata.org/life-expectancy.

9. Dan Buettner and Sam Skemp, "Blue Zones: Lessons from the World's Longest Lived," *American Journal of Lifestyle Medicine* 10, no. 5 (2016): 318–21, https:// pubmed.ncbi.nlm.nih.gov/30202288/.

10. Marion Nestle, *Food Politics: How the Food Industry Influences Nutrition and Health* (Berkeley: University of California Press, 2013), 7.

11. Donald C. Willcox, Giovanni Scapagnini, and Bradley J. Willcox, "Healthy Aging Diets Other than the Mediterranean: A Focus on the Okinawan Diet," *Mechanisms of Ageing and Development* 136 (2014): 148–62, https://pubmed.ncbi.nlm.nih.gov/24462788/.

12. Barry M. Popkin, "The Nutrition Transition and Its Health Implications in Lower-Income Countries," *Public Health Nutrition* 1, no. 1 (1998): 5–21, https://pubmed.ncbi.nlm.nih.gov/10555527/.

CONCLUSION: TRADE-OFFS IN THE FUTURE OF FOOD

1. Yinon M. Bar-On, Rob Phillips, and Ron Milo, "The Biomass Distribution on Earth," *PNAS (Proceedings of the National Academy of Sciences)*, April 13, 2018, pnas.org/doi/10.1073/pnas.1711842115.

2. H. Charles J. Godfray, Paul Aveyard, Tara Garnett, Jim H. Hall, Timothy J. Key, Jamie Lorimer, Ray T. Pierrehumbert, Peter Scarborough, Marco Springmann, and Susan A. Jebb, "Meat Consumption, Health, and the Environment," *Science* 361, no. 6399 (2018), https://science.org/doi/10.1126/science.aam5324.

3. Philip H. Howard, Francesco Ajena, Marina Yamaoka, and Amber Clarke, " 'Protein' Industry Convergence and its Implications for Resilient and Equitable Food Systems," *Frontiers in Sustainable Food Systems* (2021), https://frontiersin.org/articles/10.3389/fsufs.2021.684181/full.

4. Peter Newton and Daniel Blaustein-Rejto, "Social and Economic Opportunities and Challenges of Plant-Based and Cultured Meat for Rural Producers in the US," *Frontiers in Sustainable Food Syst*ems (2021), https://frontiersin.org/articles/10.3389/fsufs.2021.624270/full.

5. Garrett M. Broad, "Plant-Based and Cell-Based Animal Product Alternatives: An Assessment and Agenda for Food Tech Justice" *Geoforum* 107 (2019): 223–226, https://www.sciencedirect.com/science/article/abs/pii/S0016718519302015.

6. Cara C. MacInnis and Gordon Hodson, "It Ain't Easy Eating Greens: Evidence of Bias Toward Vegetarians and Vegans from Both Source and Target," *Group Processes and Intergroup Relations* 20, no. 6 (2015): 721–44, https://journals.sagepub.com/doi/10.1177/1368430215618253.

7. Ibid.

8. Matthew Cole and Karen Morgan, "Vegaphobia: Derogatory Discourses of Veganism and the Reproduction of Speciesism in UK National Newspapers," *British Journal of Sociology* 62, no. 1 (2011): 134–53, https://onlinelibrary.wiley.com/doi/abs/10.1111/j.1468-4446.2010.01348.x.

9. Alex Berke and Kent Larson, "The Negative Impact of Vegetarian and Vegan Labels: Results from Randomized Controlled Experiments with US Consumers," *Appetite* 118 (2023): 106767, https://sciencedirect.com/science/article/pii/S0195666323017476.

10. Faunalytics, "A Summary of Faunalytics' Study of Current and Former Vegetarians and Vegans," February 2016, https://faunalytics.org/a-summary-of-faunalytics-study-of-current-and-former-vegetarians-and-vegans/.

11. J. Wood, "Costa Rica Has Doubled Its Tropical Rainforests in Just a Few Decades. Here's How," *World Economic Forum*, June 13, 2019, https://weforum.org/agenda/2019/06/costa-rica-has-doubled-its-tropical-rainforests-in-just-a-few-decades-here-s-how.

12. Douglas Guilbeault and Damon Centola, "Topological Measures for Identifying and Predicting the Spread of Complex Contagions," *Nature Communications* 12, no. 4430 (2021): 1–9, https://www.nature.com/articles/s41467-021-24704-6.

13. Joseph Poore and Thomas Nemecek, "Reducing Food's Environmental Impacts Through Producers and Consumers," *Science* 360, no. 6392 (2018): 987–92, https://www.science.org/doi/10.1126/science.aaq0216.

14. Arjen Y. Hoekstra and Mesfin M. Mekonnen, "The Water Footprint of Humanity," *Proceedings of the National Academy of Sciences* 109, no. 9 (2012): 3232–37, https://www.pnas.org/doi/full/10.1073/pnas.1109936109.

15. Walter Sullivan, "The Einstein Papers. A Man of Many Parts," *New York Times*, March 29, 1972, https://nytimes.com/1972/03/29/archives/the-einstein-papers-a-man-of-many-parts-the-einstein-papers-man-of.html.

INDEX

A NOTE ON THE AUTHOR

NINA GUILBEAULT (née Gheihman) is cofounder of Plant Futures, and previously a postdoctoral scholar at the Sustainable Food Initiative at the University of California, Berkeley. Her work has been covered by the *Atlantic*, the *Telegraph*, and *Refinery29*. The coauthor of *Habits of Inequality*, she holds a doctorate in sociology from Harvard University and a certificate of plant-based nutrition from the T. Colin Campbell Center for Nutrition Studies. She lives in Berkeley.